INSATIABLE
WIVES

INSATIABLE WIVES

WOMEN WHO STRAY
AND THE MEN WHO
LOVE THEM

DAVID J. LEY

ROWMAN & LITTLEFIELD PUBLISHERS, INC.
Lanham • Boulder • New York • Toronto • Plymouth, UK

Published by Rowman & Littlefield Publishers, Inc.
A wholly owned subsidiary of The Rowman & Littlefield Publishing Group, Inc.
4501 Forbes Boulevard, Suite 200, Lanham, Maryland 20706
www.rowmanlittlefield.com

Estover Road, Plymouth PL6 7PY, United Kingdom

British Library Cataloguing in Publication Information Available

Library of Congress Cataloging-in-Publication Data

Ley, David J., 1973–
    Insatiable wives : women who stray and the men who love them /
  David J. Ley
      p. cm.
    Includes bibliographical references and index.
    ISBN 978-1-4422-0030-2 (cloth : alk. paper) —
    ISBN 978-1-4422-0032-6 (electronic)
    1. Married women—Sexual behavior. 2. Wives—Sexual behavior.
3. Promiscuity. I. Title.
HQ29.L488 2009
306.77086'550973—dc22   2009020211

∞™ The paper used in this publication meets the minimum requirements of
American National Standard for Information Sciences—Permanence of Paper
for Printed Library Materials, ANSI/NISO Z39.48-1992.

Printed in the United States of America

This work is dedicated to my wife, who taught me the meaning of love. Without her, I would be a lesser man, living a smaller life.

CONTENTS

CONTENTS

ACKNOWLEDGMENTS

First and foremost, I must acknowledge the couples and individuals who shared with me their most private thoughts, fantasies, and behaviors. Without their warmth, openness, and trust, this book could not have been written.

The support of many people was essential in the creation of this book. Angela Kilman was a dear friend and first reader. All of my friends and colleagues were patient and supportive with me, as I discussed the sometimes shocking and titillating contents of my book and investigations. Thanks for listening.

Fellow psychologists, therapists, and researchers were tremendously helpful, and include too many folks to name, but Dr. Steven Gangestad, Dr. Uri Wernik, and Dr. Marty Klein deserve special recognition for their personal support. Tony Dipasquale was involved from the beginning, and brought a wealth of support and understanding to my project.

My employer, River Valley Consulting, deserves special acknowledgment for providing me a wonderful career and opportunity to develop professionally.

The experience of publishing was made extremely easy and painless for me—a first-time writer—by my agent, Mike Hamilburg, and my editor at Rowman & Littlefield, Suzanne Staszak-Silva. Extra thanks go to writer John C. Waugh, for his assistance and encouragement in entering the publishing process.

INTRODUCTION

I first encountered what is called "the hotwife phenomenon" in 2005, while collecting e-mail responses for a research study surveying couples on the Internet. Two respondents described their participation in what they called the "hotwife lifestyle," and offered descriptions of the wife's sexual promiscuity, with the full support and encouragement of the husband. One of the women was a corporate executive with a personal salary well into six figures. She had lived this lifestyle for many years and described a history of literally hundreds of different male sex partners, all with the explicit support and encouragement of her monogamous husband.

At first disbelieving, I assumed that this was akin to an urban legend, a phenomenon that existed solely in the fantasies of some males, as they used the Internet to wildly exaggerate the Madonna–whore image of their wives. But a few Internet searches revealed numerous sites dedicated to the discussion and celebration of hotwives, and led to the suspicion that there was far more to the story. And yet, despite the growing presence and long history of this subculture, there is incredibly little mainstream attention to it.

Kai Ma published *Take My Wife, Please*, on the website Nerve.com. The article is one of the very few in the popular press, addressing this lifestyle. It discussed the phenomenon of hotwives, and introduced a couple and one of the men with whom the wife had sex, while the husband filmed. I was intrigued by the article's premise; these were normal people. Healthy and successful people. These weren't marriages that were "on the rocks," where permissive infidelity was a last ditch effort to save the marriage. Many of the couples living this lifestyle were successful, often highly educated people. These were folks I expected to see in college classrooms or around business boardroom tables. I didn't expect rampant sexual promiscuity, and a celebration of female sexual infidelity in such couples.

When I talked about this to friends, colleagues, and even acquaintances, once I got past their strange and suspicious looks, I found I wasn't alone in my disbelief. Universally, people responded with the belief that such a lifestyle was bound to destroy a marriage, a husband's self-esteem, and couldn't possibly, in any way, shape, or form, be a healthy part of a married couple's sexual life. Certainly, people who chose this lifestyle could only be doing so out of deep-seated pathologies, character flaws, and histories of sexual trauma and abandonment. The very few people who didn't respond with such automatic assumptions revealed that they had kinks of their own, which had led them to develop "broader opinions about what is and isn't healthy."

Researchers have explored the perceptions held by therapists regarding marital relationships that are not monogamous, by agreement within the couple. Therapists, psychiatrists, and others in the helping professions view such relationships as inherently dysfunctional and emerging from deep-seated psychopathology and personality disturbance. These viewpoints still persist, despite the increasing occurrence and awareness of nonmonogamous relationships. Many polyamorous and swinging couples have expressed distrust and resentment toward revealing their lifestyle and details of their sexual practices, due to stigma and judgment from society.

The couples I encountered encouraged me to explore this phenomenon further. It struck me how wrong my base assumptions might be, and how those erroneous assumptions could affect my own clinical work. If I held such assumptions, and couples that practiced this lifestyle entered my office, would they tell me? Would I allow them to tell me? At this point, I frankly suspect they would not, and that chances are good I've had clients who did not disclose their interests in this lifestyle. How is it that the field of health care is so conflicted about this lifestyle that most couples simply refrain from disclosure? How is it that these couples are out there living a lifestyle that is so contrary to core assumptions about love, sexuality, monogamy, and fidelity? Why also are those core assumptions out there? Is this a new lifestyle, fueled by the Internet, or is this something that has been around as long as marriage, and if so, why is it such a secret?

I set out to interview some of these couples, and attempt a beginning description of this lifestyle, and the people who choose it, using an online personals site, Craigslist, where a good many of these couples arrange their extramarital sexual adventures. These interviews can represent only a sample, and a biased sample at that, of the couples who pursue this lifestyle. The interviews I present in interludes after each chapter are only those of couples who chose to respond to my advertisements. I made an effort to present as broad and varied a view as possible, both in recruiting couples, and in the interviews I chose to include. I scoured academic and general literature, to try to understand the various issues involved in these couples' lives. Many couples and individuals directed me to writings they had found, that addressed these issues, however obliquely.

Along the way, my questions grew. Each answer raised more questions. Each query led my research, my questions, and my potential answers, into growing and expanding areas of history, science, and research. In order to understand these couples and their sexual choices, I found I had to understand monogamy, as well as its alternatives. As I realized that these couples celebrated an unrestrained female sexuality, I had to gain some understanding of where, how, and why female sexuality was constrained in our society and history. As they celebrated female sexuality, I found that I had to learn better what female sexuality was, for each individual woman, and for humankind at large. At last, I found that to understand why these couples did what they did, I had to gain some understanding of what the role and effects of sexuality and mating were, both within the body and mind, and within the evolutionary history of humans. As I present some of my answers and questions along the way, I cannot offer the full wealth or context of these fields and endeavors. I was blessed to find many authors and researchers who had a far greater understanding of the depths of these fields than I will ever possess. The research and findings, the history and events that I present represent only the smallest portion of the wealth of information out there about each of these topics. I make no effort to present the full history of female sexuality. Such a work, truly a noble endeavor, would take a lifetime. Instead, I present the facts and findings that most helped me to develop some understanding of why and how these couples do what they do, and why their behavior came as such a surprise to me.

As blessed as I was to find a wealth of written information about sexuality, and the writers and researchers who compiled this information, I was even luckier to find people who were willing to share their lives and choices with me. Men and women, husbands and wives, who were willing to sit with me and explain who they were and how they came to make the choices they've made. In person and on the phone, via e-mail and Internet posts, these people were willing to help me understand. At first, many of them were suspicious. For some, their suspicion never went away. They were fearful that I was on a quest to label them and others like them, to point them out as sick or perverted, to brand them with the scarlet letter of adultery. Many of them believed my questions and research were a ploy, a fraud, perpetrated to create situations in which I could seek illicit sex. But, those who were willing opened themselves up to me, and showed me their lives and marriages, for all that they are, good and bad, so that I could understand them, their lives, and their choices.

There is a huge Internet following of wife sharing, hotwifing, and cuckoldry. Hundreds of thousands of Internet sites exist, dedicated to the celebration of these lifestyles. I could not ever visit all of them. Early on, a couple with whom I corresponded directed me to the site OurHotwives.org. There are many sites out there like this one, where husbands, wives, and couples exhaustively discuss and share the intricacies of their sexual lives and choices. But, the moderator and members of this website were accepting of my questions, and responsive to my thoughts. As I had questions about one or another issue that emerged along the way, the members of this site were willing to share their thoughts and experiences. Sprinkled throughout this book are quotes from these members, as they were relevant to the topic at hand.

In the cases of both the interviews and e-mail/Internet forum quotes I present, I have done my best to both protect the confidentiality of the individuals and couples, and preserve the spirit and truth of their words. I have changed names, and in many cases, I have blended the words and stories of different people. Sometimes, I have used one couple's story to present the words and experiences of many others. Any errors are my own. I have endeavored to present these stories and lives with respect, and to honor these people, and their marriages.

In offering quotes and stories of these people, I have tried to offer to you the reader, the same experience I had, of encountering these people, these husbands and wives, in their own words, in their own lives. I choose to follow the choice of Andrew, whose story is told in the first interlude. He defines his and his wife's activities as "sharing." Among swingers, the term "wife swapping" fell out of favor, as it implied the wife was an object to be "swapped" with other men, like a trade item. An element of this objectification is still present in the term sharing, but there is a much stronger core meaning of cooperation, union, relationship, and communication, implicit in the idea of sharing. Robert Heinlein, who explored nonmonogamous relationships in many of his books, had characters who "shared water," as a symbolic gesture of joining with others, and melding one's life with another. Likewise, these couples choose to share the wife's sexuality with others, in a way that strengthens the bonds between husband and wife, and sometimes, between them and other men.

1

BIRDS AND HORNS

Spring (and love) is in the air. Birds chirp amidst the trees, darting between the slender branches. It is that time when flowers bloom, bees buzz, and babies are born, with the long spring and summer before them. Amidst the stiff, green-tipped reeds along a marshy river bank, a nest of twigs is built by a small female reed warbler and her mate. The birds, light brown in color, gather twigs and blades of grass, weaving them into a basket, tucked inside a small bush. As the birds work, they are unaware that they are being watched. In the trees, hidden by the leaves, is another female bird. Slightly larger than the reed warbler, with a yellowish bill, the female *cuculus canorus* watches intently as the warblers build their nest. This bird's mate is off hunting insects to eat, and that night, they will share their own nest. Their nest is considerably smaller than the one the warblers are building, sort of a "honeymoon cottage," compared to the "starter family home" the warblers are crafting.

Weeks pass as the warblers complete their nest. At last, the female warbler squats in their basket of twigs, her wings spread, and deposits a clutch of small eggs in the protected bower. Her labor complete, she leaves the eggs unguarded and flies off to feed. The female stalker swoops in. She deftly places her yellow bill against one of the small eggs, and strains her small legs and body, pushing the egg up and over the side of the nest. It disappears amidst the debris that covers the marshy ground beneath the bush. How this female knew that the warbler had at last laid her clutch, no one knows. But she did, and now the job of egg-removal complete, the female squats in the nest and delivers her own egg amidst the others. Similar in shape and size, it blends in. She deposits only one, and then flies away without a single look back. She visits several nests that day, as other warblers leave their new eggs alone and unguarded. She'll lay no eggs in her own nest, nor will she worry about feeding any squalling young birds in the months to come.

The warblers return home, finding nothing amiss. The small brown female nestles against the eggs, sharing the warmth of her body. Weeks pass, and one of the eggs shakes, trembling, as a small head bursts forth. The female, enraptured by the first birth of her brood, fails to notice that the baby's bill is much lighter in color than her own. The chick grows rapidly, while the other eggs have not yet hatched. Indeed, each day, there are fewer eggs in the nest, though still only one baby chick, demanding food. When the warblers are away, you see, the baby chick imitates his mother, putting his back against an egg, and shoving it out of the nest, where it joins that first egg, lost in the mud.

At last, a few of the warblers' remaining eggs do hatch, their inhabitants crawling out into the nest. Their older foster brother is less than overjoyed to see them. When the warblers' return home, their mouths full of bugs, he overpowers the younger birds, seizing the food before they can. Starving, they become even weaker, and offer little resistance when he pushes them out of the nest. Falling to the mud, they are quick prey to snakes, bugs, and the soft, marshy earth, their plaintive cries lost to the louder "goo-koos" of their foster brother. After a bit more than six weeks, only he remains in the nest, fed by the dedicated warbler parents. One day, he too flies off, without a look back, just like his mother, to find his own mate, who will one day deposit their own eggs amidst the nests of other unsuspecting warblers.

Postscript: Sadly, the reed warblers are not quite the monogamous, innocent victims this avian couple might appear. Prior to the cuckoo's visit, there were many other illicit visitors in this couple's nest. Male warblers visited the nest to copulate with the female, leaving just before her mate returned home. Many of the eggs rolled out of the nest by the cuckoo were not fathered by the male of this mated pair. And where is the male returning from? From the nest of yet other warbler mating pairs, where he has also gone visiting, leaving his genes in other nests, as a strategy to increase the likelihood that somewhere, in some nest, his children will survive.

The fear, for men experiencing wives having sex with other men, is that the husband may unknowingly rear the children of another man, and his own children might lose out to the children of this other, unknown male. As with the chicks of a nest co-opted by a cuckoo, the child of another man, born to one's wife, might use up valuable family and parental resources, depriving other children. That other father must be quite sneaky, appealing, or seductive, in order to steal the willing pleasures of one's wife, and thus, his child may also come into a man's nest with skills of seduction that the husband's own children lack.

Cuckoldry, and the social response to it, has a long, complex, and mostly dark history in man. Sexual jealousy and possessiveness, with violent, often deadly consequences, is present among every human culture. Even those cultures believed to be more sexually permissive, still punished female adultery, usually in violent fashion. Some rare cultures allowed, even celebrated female sexual infidelity, making it an important part of family and social function. Today, increasing numbers of couples are exploring a lifestyle they call "hotwifing" or "cuckoldry," where the couple's sexual activity centers upon an exploration of the wife's sexual encounters with other men. This lifestyle represents a remarkable deviation from the long history of social punishment and prohibition of cuckoldry, ostensibly intended to limit the chances of a man unknowingly raising the children of another man.

> Cuckoldry is a reproductive cost inflicted on a man by a woman's sexual infidelity or temporary defection from her regular long-term relationship . . . These costs include loss of the time, effort, and resources the man has spent attracting his partner, the potential misdirection of his resources to his rival's offspring, and the loss of his mate's investment in offspring he may have had with her in the future.[1]

> The unfaithfulness of the wife, as compared with that of the husband, is morally of much wider bearing, and should always meet with severer punishment at the hands of the law. The unfaithful wife not only dishonours herself, but also her husband and her family, not to speak of the possible uncertainty of paternity.[2]

The word *cuckold*, by most accounts, emerges from the habits of the cuckoo bird. Some cuckoo birds have evolved a reproductive strategy, whereby the female secretly lays her eggs in the nests of other birds, which then unknowingly care for the eggs and raise the cuckoo's fledglings as their own. The cuckoo bird, of which there are many species, seems an unlikely target to inspire such fear and anger as emerges around the fear of being cuckolded. Most species of the *cuculidae* bird family are small, inoffensive birds. The coccyx, the human tailbone, was named after the cuckoo, because the Greeks saw a resemblance between the wedge-shaped bone at the base of the spine, and the cuckoo's bill. In England, the call of the cuckoo is regarded as the first sign of spring, and in Russia, there is legend that, if asked, the cuckoo can tell a man how many years he will live. Not all of the cuckoo species are what biologists term "brood parasites," in that only some species of the bird practice the deceptive act of laying their eggs in the nests of birds whose eggs resemble their own. The cuckoo is a pretty sly bird, and tends to keep a low profile. Funnily enough, the cuckoo is, in many cases, a monogamous species, establishing long-term mates. I wonder though, does the male cuckoo ever wonder why he doesn't have any kids like other birds do? Or does he just breathe a sigh of relief, wipe his feathered brow, and thank God for resourceful mates?

In a 1938 *Time* magazine, the record of a divorce case contains a fascinating tale of cuckoldry. A "Negro maid," testified in a Brooklyn, New York, divorce case about the infidelity of her employer's wife.[3] What is extraordinary about this incident is that instead of describing the wife's covert activities, her sneaking in and out of the home, and her secret male lover, the maid accused the wife using no words. She quietly put her hand on her forehead, raising two fingers like horns, in a symbol called "cornuto," nonverbally accusing her employer's wife of sexual infidelity. This Italian traditional symbol for cuckold emerged from the practice of grafting spurs (cut from the bird's feet) onto the heads of castrated fighting cocks (roosters that is). Thus, by using the horns as a symbol for a cuckold, the assertion is that this man is really not manly at all, like the castrated cockerel.

These horns, and other metaphorical and symbolic discussions of cuckoldry arise through much great literature of European history. During the Jacobite movement in eighteenth-century Britain, effigies of King George I were often burned, with horns attached to his head. (George and his wife Sophia had separated, each taking lovers. Eventually, Sophia's lover, a Swedish count, was killed, and Sophia imprisoned for the remainder of her life, to prevent the scandal of her affair from tainting the monarchy and the King.)

Other early works of literature carry similar fears and derisive comments about cuckolds, often with references to the horns that symbolize a cuckold. In *The Merry Wives of Windsor*, act II, scene II, Falstaff says:

> Hang him, poor cuckoldly knave! I know him not: yet I wrong him to call him poor; they say the jealous wittolly knave hath masses of money; for the which his wife seems to me well-favored. I will use her as the key of the cuckoldly rogue's coffer; and there's my harvest-home.

He continues, describing his plans to use cuckolding as a way to steal Ford's money:

> I will stare him out of his wits; I will awe him with my cudgel: it shall hang like a meteor o'er the cuckold's horns. Master Brook, thou shalt know I will predominate over the peasant, and thou shalt lie with his wife. Come to me soon at night. Ford's a knave, and I will aggravate his style; thou, Master Brook, shalt know him for knave and cuckold. Come to me soon at night.

In Shakespeare, and in most history, there is little humor, and a great deal of fear, anguish, and anger with regards to cuckolding. Cuckoldry, as a tragic theme, runs through a great many of Shakespearean works, including most notably the tragedy of *Othello*. Driven by fear of being cuckolded, Othello is led to believe that wife Desdemona has cuckolded him with his friend Cassio. The devious Iago feeds this fear, for his own political gain. Othello is unable to bear the thought of his wife having a secret love for Cassio, and at last suffocates the innocent Desdemona, refusing to believe her protestations of fidelity.

In *Much Ado About Nothing*, act I, scene 1, line 252, Benedick describes his fear and revulsion of cuckoldry, saying, "The savage bull may, but if ever the sensible Benedick bear it, pluck off the bull's horns and set them in my forehead." According to some folklorists, this metaphor relates to the belief that a cuckolded man had horns on his head that were invisible to him, but seen by everyone else as a badge of his public shame and insufficiency in his marriage. This idea of "invisibility" seems to emerge from the idea that when a woman is cheating on her husband, he is usually the last person in the community to know, as everyone is whispering around him, and his friends are drawing straws over which one will be the one to tell him. Males through history who are cuckolded have experienced social humiliation, the derision, and, ostensibly, the shame that comes with that social experience. The implicit social assumption is that a "real man" is expected to be able to either satisfy his wife such that she has no need of other men, or that he can exert such fear and control over her, that she would never allow or pursue sex outside their marriage. Sometimes, stories of cuckolded husbands appear to have been fabricated by other men, in order to "bring down" powerful men in government and society. English taverns were full of men who boasted of sex with the wives of judges and government officials, making powerful men appear not powerful enough to either satisfy or control their wives. Many cultures and languages have terms to describe the unfortunate male, who unknowingly raises the child of another man. In English, the word is "cuckold," ostensibly derived from the cuckoo, and its "gookoo" call. In Chinese, it is "*dài l mà*," which reportedly means, "wears a green hat." Few Chinese men wear green hats, as you can imagine. Indeed, foreigners are cautioned not to give a Chinese friend a gift of a green hat, as he may assume that you are offering him a quiet nudge that his wife or girlfriend has another lover.

"Cabron," in Spanish, labels a male as being like a goat, who has given up his masculinity. Notably, the term cabron is often applied to men who know about their wives' infidelity, and lack the "manhood," or the cojones one supposes, to do anything about it. "Wittol" is a similar term from Middle English, describing the cuckold that is aware of his wife's infidelity, and does nothing. The word is supposedly derived from the term "witting cuckold," as in a "knowing" cuckold. UrbanDictionary.com defines wittol similarly, and exemplifies the meaning with the following use in a sentence: "When his wife told him she had just made love to his best friend, her husband, being a wittol, wished her happiness, and his wife displayed appropriate affectionate contempt for her husband."[4] In current usage among the cuckold and hotwife communities, however, the term cuckold is used to describe the man that knows about his wife's extramarital sexual encounters, and indeed, celebrates them.

In Brazil, researcher Claudia Fonseca found that the assumption that Latin American male machismo would create dramatic fear and anger towards cuckoldry was largely untrue. In Brazilian culture, the archetypes of women are often divided into only two images, "santa" (the good mother and wife), or the "piranha" (the promiscuous, sexually voracious woman).[5] But, in the working-class neighborhoods she investigated, Fonseca found that another term was often applied to women, particularly women who "got away with" adultery. They were called "malandra," or "wily woman." These women were able to establish their husbands in the role of a "corno manso," or a compliant cuckold.

Sometimes, men were punished publicly and informally for their wives' cuckoldry of them, and were made to "ride skimmington." This tradition began as a means to ridicule men who allowed their wives to beat them, often with a ladle called a "skimmington." The town would have a parade, placing the man backward on a horse, while women beat him with a giant fake skimmington, and other townsfolk blew horns and beat frying pans. When the man who rode skimmington was a cuckold, bull's horns were added to the melee, and sometimes even tied to the cuckold's forehead. In France, a similar community response to cuckoldry was called "charivari." Charivari is also the term used for public shaming of husbands in Brazil, a custom still common in working-class and poverty-stricken areas of the country.

The cuckolding men, who frisked with wives of other men, were also sometimes the recipients of punishment. They were sometimes "carted," or tied to the wheel of a cart and whipped. One such man famously received his lashings from a girdle, after he was discovered with another man's wife. No word on whether the girdle that was wielded belonged to the wife or not. In Colonial America, a man caught with another man's wife might be banished, or even, on one occasion, was made to stand in the square with a noose around his neck, for the entire village to see.

In Asia, men who were caught in sexual relations with another man's wife were punished severely, as the adulterous act brought dishonor upon the husband's entire family. As a result, these men could face gruesome death, sometimes by burning, or suicide if they were lucky. In India, a man caught with a guru's wife could be forced to sit upon a heated iron plate, and then compelled to use a knife to sever his own penis. (There were not a lot of repeat offenders, one can assume.)

Peter the Great, czar of Russia, upon discovering his wife's infidelity had her lover decapitated. The man's head was preserved in a jar of alcohol and kept in the bedroom of Peter's wife, upon his orders. Apparently, the Russians have a thing for jars—after his death, Rasputin, known for his sexual escapades with many society wives, including Czarina Alexandra, was castrated. His penis, alleged to be over eleven inches long, is reportedly preserved in a jar and available for viewing in a St. Petersburg museum of erotica, run by the chief of prostate research at the Russian Academy of Natural Sciences.

But, the real punishment for cuckolding falls most heavily upon the wife. One of the first known tales of female adultery appears in Egyptian legends dating from around 2600 BC, about the Pharaoh Nabka and the wife of a man named Ubau-anir. One of the Pharaoh's royal vassals was apparently very attracted to Ubau-anir's wife, who invited him to lay with her in her gardens. They did, and then the wife conspired with him to arrange a retreat to one of her husband's properties on the shore of a lake. Unfortunately, the overseer of the property reported the wife's plans to her husband. Ubau-anir used sorcery to kill his wife's lover, creating a magical crocodile that killed him while the lover was on a moonlight swim. Then, at the Pharaoh's direction, the husband burned his wife alive, throwing her ashes in the river. Given the Egyptian belief in the need for mummification to preserve one's body for the afterlife, a death in such a manner was the equivalent of not only death in this life, but prevention of ever entering any afterlife as well.

In Europe, particularly in Germany, women discovered in extramarital sex, or even suspected of infidelity, were punished severely, often with death. Adulterous women had their heads shaved by their husbands, were stripped before the town, beaten and flogged as they were driven from their village. Adulterous women were stoned to death, burned, hanged, and drowned. In a ceremony that was co-opted for other purposes during witch trials, the Franks tied a stone around an adulterous woman's neck and cast her in the water. If she survived, she was innocent. These German traditional values remained strong. Nineteenth-century German eugenicist Max Gruber described female chastity as a great national possession, which was essential to support healthy families, and a healthy society. He suggested that this was the reason men fought against female infidelity, not mere sexual selfishness, but because female sexual infidelity had the potential of destroying the fabric of German society.

Sicily, in the twelfth century, passed laws that prohibited execution, but did confiscate the property of the man who slept with another man's wife, and ordered that the nose of the unfaithful wife be slit as a sign of her infidelity. In Samoa, a cuckolded husband would actually bite off the nose of the unfaithful wife. In India, both the nose, and the clitoris of an unfaithful wife were severed. Roman law allowed a man to simply, and immediately, kill a wife whom he caught in infidelity (though for some period of Roman rule, the husband did only have sixty days to punish the wife. If sixty days without punishment passed after he found out about her infidelity, she was apparently off the hook). In some cases, they were also drowned or thrown into bogs to die a slow death. Such was the recorded fate of Queen Gunnhild, known as the Scandinavian "Mother of Kings."

Gunnhild konungamóir lived in tenth-century Scandinavia, born to the king of Denmark. She later married Erik the Bloodax, king of Norway. Many of her children went on to rule Norway, and she is a prominent figure in Norwegian legend and history. Gunnhild, alleged to have magical powers of witchcraft (which appear to have actually been very savvy political skills) cut a memorable swath through the halls of power in Scandinavia, advising (and killing) political leaders throughout the region. After her husband Erik died, she continued her political influence and involvement, through her sons and through her own relationships. She took on a lover, a chieftain named Hrut, who she ultimately used her magic to curse with priapism (a clinical condition resulting in a painful, unyielding, and unresolving erection) when Hrut married another woman. There are hints that Gunnhild used her sexuality throughout her life to control and influence men around her. After eventually returning to Denmark, Gunnhild was killed by a former political partner (and possibly bedmate), King Harald Bluetooth. She was slain in the manner traditional for unfaithful women, drowned in a bog. In the 1800s, the mummified body of a woman killed in that manner was recovered from a bog in Jutland,

and was reburied in a grand sarcophagus by the king of Denmark, under the (mistaken) belief this was the body of Gunnhild. Sadly, it was not, and was later established to be the body of some other poor woman, killed in a bog, probably for infidelity, hundreds of years before the life and death of Queen Gunnhild.

Colonial America was not free of these practices. In Massachusetts, in 1643, young colonist Mary Latham reportedly fell in love with a man who spurned her love. Rejected, Mary married a much, much older man. Predictably, Mary did not remain spurned by men her own age for long, nor did her fickle commitment to her husband persist for long. Fights began with her husband, as young men in the colony began to seek her favors. In one fight, she threatened her elderly husband with a knife, calling him a "cuckold," and threatening to kill him. One morning, colonists discovered Mary lying intoxicated and unclothed on the ground, with one of her suitors, James Britton. She was found guilty, and sentenced to death, along with young Mr. Britton. They were hanged together on March 21. This case was an exception to the rule; in Britain and America, execution was only levied against infidelity in a few, rare cases.

In this instance, American law is quite different from the earliest biblical law, where only the woman was held responsible and punished for adultery. Though the commandment does say they shall not covet their neighbor's wife, slaves, donkey, or possessions, men were rarely, if ever, punished for sampling the grass on the other side of the fence. In Hebraic tradition, men were commanded to ensure their wives were satisfied. To give one's wife sexual satisfaction was considered mitzvah, or a sacred, and necessary, act of kindness. Rabbis set sexual expectations based upon the husband's social status, whereby peasants could have sex weekly, though academics and learned men were to only have sex once in two years. When they did have sex, the man was encouraged to satisfy his wife. But, it was not acceptable for that academic's unsatisfied wife to seek mitzvah from some other kind-hearted man.

In Deuteronomy, the adulterous wife is condemned to death by stoning and cursed to a bloated, rotting death in Numbers. In Jewish law, a man could divorce his wife, simply by writing a "bill of divorce," arranging for two witnesses (presumably male witnesses), and giving it to her. Similarly, in Arabic traditions, a cuckolded husband had only to say "I divorce thee," using the formal Arabic word "Taliq" with two witnesses present. There is specific Muslim attention to cases where a man may have sex with the wife of another man, such that he divorces her, and she marries her lover. This divorce and remarriage are legal, and allowable, though Islamic law notes that both man and woman have committed significant sin.

However, in the New Testament, Christ extends this condemnation of infidelity, now to include the husband. Marriage is a sacred bond, like unto the bond between man and God, and "What God hath joined together, let no man put asunder" (Mark 10:9). Even further, the man who divorces his wife and marries another woman is committing the sin of adultery (Mark 10:11). In the Book of John, the adulterous woman, to be stoned to death in accord with Deuteronomy, is saved by Christ, who asks that only that person without sin be the first to throw a stone. Thus, adultery, while a sin, is now held even with other sins, and is a commandment for both man and woman.

In eighteenth-century Europe, numerous texts were published that warned against female adultery. The popular works claimed that sex by wives with men other than their husband led to the birth of crippled and deformed offspring, and could render a wife sterile and incapable of producing an heir for the husband, invoking and stoking the fires that fed evolutionary pressures on male reproduction and supported the fears of cuckoldry. Female infidelity was typically regarded as far more significant than male infidelity.

In England, cuckoldry was not uncommon, even among the lower classes. In fact, cuckoldry was sometimes arranged by a husband and wife, as a way to extort money from the wife's lover. Divorce was granted only by the English government, and rarely at that, but civil trials for damages were common. "Wounded" husbands were often awarded significant financial settlements by the courts, moneys owed by the male lover to the husband. Theophilus Cibber and his wife Susannah Maria apparently attempted such a scheme in the eighteenth century, attempting to earn an award of five thousand pounds from a Mr. Sloper for his sexual encounter with Susannah Maria. Unfortunately, the jury felt that Cibber and his wife had arranged the adulterous encounter, intending to entrap Mr. Sloper with the purpose of financial reward, and returned a verdict that awarded Cibber no damages.

Financial gain was one significant reason husbands shared their wives. According to seventeenth-century writer Seignur de Brantome, one husband from Ferrara used his wife in an "abominable and despicable" manner.[6] According to Brantome, this husband had pursued a young man for some time, though the young man rejected the husband's sexual advances. At last, knowing that the young man desired his wife, the husband arranged with his wife for her to seduce the young man. In the midst of their encounter, the husband entered the bedchamber, acted surprised, and threatened the young man with death, which was his right according to Italian law. As an alternative, the husband offered to change places with his wife. According to the translation by Zacks, Brantome wrote "Thus was the husband [willingly] cuckolded in an extremely vile way."[7]

Mary Combes was a seventeenth-century innkeeper's wife in Somerset, England, whose loud, public cuckoldry was known to the entire county. Mary's story is recounted by G. R. Quaife, in his analysis of sexuality in English court records. Mary was infamously sexual with almost any man she could lay hands upon. In their inn, male drinkers reported that after delivering their ale, Mary would grab their crotches and tell the man, "if it were ready to stand, she was ready for him."[8] One man, who reportedly had trouble with impotence, was ridiculed by Mary, who claimed she had brought starch, and intended to use it "to make it stand" for her.[9] Mary lay in the crossroads at times, spreading her legs to male travelers, calling out "Come play with [me] and make my husband a cuckold."[10] Mary would proudly parade through town in the nude, and any man she found lying on his back in front of her could expect her to lift her skirts (if she were wearing any) and plop herself down onto his crotch. She was accused of "indecently forcing honest men to occupy her," by "spreading her legs abroad and showing her commodity."[11] In 1653, this innkeeper's wife held a party, an alcohol-fueled orgy, that she proclaimed was "only for cuckolds and cuckold-makers."[12] Mary Combes was brought before the county legal system many times for her lewdness, but her husband and neighbors always defended her, and she was never punished.

In England, men caught with other men's wives sometimes made initial offers of six to eight pennies, accepting that the wounded husband would bargain him up to as much as twenty to forty shillings, in order to forget that the other man had been caught with one's wife.

Sometimes, wives were shared with other men, in order to secure other economic services. In Dunster, Owen Howe and his wife found an elderly, wealthy man, to whom they attached themselves, his wife having sex with the man, while Owen bled him dry of his finances. Attewell Leiker, of Asholt, England, found several young men who were looking for lodging, inviting them, at various times to live with he and his wife. Once ensconced in their home, Attewell invited them into his bed with he and his wife, Elizabeth. Attewell encouraged the man to sleep next to Elizabeth, who then took over, using "inticing words and impudent behavior," using her body to seduce the men.[13] Once the men were under her control, Elizabeth then took to encouraging these young men to steal for her—from their employers and relatives—until they were apprehended and the full story emerged in court.

The "wifely whore," whose husband would pander to other men, was a relatively common fixture in many villages of the past. Among the M'pongo tribe in Gabun, wives were often rented to other men, particularly to Europeans. Children that resulted were usually raised by the family, as their own. M'pongo wives who resisted being rented out were convinced through the husband's use of a hippopotamus-skin whip. Also in Africa, the men of the Galla tribe would punish infidelity or sexual overtures toward their wives, but would willingly offer their wife if provided payment. In modern-day Nevada, many of the prostitutes working in brothels have husbands and boyfriends who send their wives to the brothels, and pocket much of the money their wives earns in bed with other men.

Sometimes, the husband didn't get away so cleanly. In one affair, recounted by Quaife, John Curtis allowed his wife to prostitute herself to James Dryall, when the couple was in financial straits. Jane continued her relationship with Dryall for seven years, as he would come to her home and they would shut themselves away in the bedroom. John Curtis didn't complain, and later stated that it was due to "the fear of mischief, shame, and the hope of amendment."[14] Finally, Jane went away with Dryall on a trip to Bristol, and upon returning, moved in with him. She took with her the Curtises' sixteen-year-old daughter, and thirteen head of their livestock. It was only then that John finally started to complain, largely because he had now been left alone in their home, with no one to cook or clean for him. Because of his long passivity, things did not go well for Curtis in court, as he tried to recover his household. Even the local judge had known for years of the scandalous lives of the Curtises and Dryall, and Curtis was chastised for only taking action when he lost livestock and a housekeeper.

Civil lawsuits in response to cuckoldry and infidelity have not disappeared. Lawsuits for "alienation of affection" still occur, even in the United States, where eight states retain such laws, allowing for tort actions against individuals who interfere in a marriage. In North Carolina, an opthalmologist was recently held liable for $200,000 in reparation to the ex-husband of his lover. Not all of the suits or penalties are filed by husbands against other men. In 1997, a Greensboro jury returned a $1 million verdict in a case for alienation of affections and criminal conversation ("criminal conversation" is legal-speak for having sex, in this context).

In 2005, Cecilia Sarkozy, former model and wife of Nicolas Sarkozy, president of France, left her husband and was photographed in New York with her new lover. Cecilia first met Sarkozy, when, in his role as mayor of Neuilly, he administered the vows she made, to her previous husband. French society was rocked by the scandal of their marital troubles, and even more stunned by Sarkozy's commitment to his wife. The couple reunited, and Sarkozy went on to continued political success. In the words of *New York Times* columnist Judith Warner, Sarkozy "transcended the old role of cuckold."[15] However, within a few short years, the couple again separated and divorced, both quickly remarrying. Critics of the French president continue to refer to his status as a cuckold, though for a man deemed ineffectual and a "classic cuckold," he continued to command substantial political power in Europe.[16]

Despite the long, long history of social prohibition and severe punishment of cuckoldry and female infidelity, it has persisted as an unspoken secret across most human societies. Some rare societies have allowed or even endorsed such practices. For the past thousand years or more, European and American societies have imposed the view that monogamy, and especially female fidelity, is the only moral, healthy, and accepted type of marital relationship. Today, those who disagree with this view have begun to assert themselves, and speak publicly about their lifestyles.

ANDREW AND MARIE

*I think it's all about attitude and physical health and we see no
end in sight. It is our way of life and we love it.*

A ndrew is a musician, his wife Marie an emeritus academic, both in
their early sixties. Andrew and Marie were the first couple I encountered who were intentionally pursuing a hotwife/cuckold lifestyle. The couple lives in the Southwest, where Andrew is retired and his wife continues
to pursue research and scholarly activities on a university campus. For several years, Andrew's wife has had a group of male lovers, with whom they
had regular threesomes, and that the wife would travel with on occasion.
Andrew is an extremely thoughtful, intelligent, and creative man, who
openly shared much of his personal story, and the history of his marriage.
Andrew was extremely open and responsive to my persistent queries, but
I was never able to interview Marie, who Andrew described as a rather private woman, despite her sexual assertiveness. She is sixty-five and he is
sixty-seven. For close to five years, Marie has had one main lover who is
in his early fifties and she also sees three "old friends" occasionally. The
couple "shares" with these other men once to twice a month.

"As numerous other people have shared, with me, and online, I also had
early deviant thoughts and feelings about sex and relationships. I think so
much of this is derived from subtle and not-so-subtle family dynamics of
how substantial topics, such as sex, were managed and the success or failure of relational aspects in the family. My earliest recollection, around age
thirteen, was of my mother getting dressed up to go to a 'meeting.' I really
don't remember what she told me, but I do remember, very clearly, my father saying to me, 'she's going to meet her lover.' He had a very sarcastic

sense of humor so I'm not assuming he meant anything special. I do recall being very excited at the idea of my mother having a lover.

"My wife grew up in the Village, in New York, with very left-wing parents. She was sexually active by age fourteen. She was also brilliant and
graduated with a doctorate in her social sciences field that allowed her substantial travel and interaction with many men at her intellectual level. She
has had an enormous number of sexual encounters. She says that she has
had 'over' two hundred lovers before I got to her. Since we married, she only
had about nine, at least . . . so far. Every once in a while, I ask her for a bed-
time story, to tell me about some of her lovers

"I met my wife when I was a single Dad, after an ugly divorce from my
first wife. I was parenting my two children, who were ten and twelve at
the time. Living where we do involves a ninety-minute commute time so
you might guess that our days were really packed with our respective professions, travel, children, household, and living in a small community with
all the expected activities, friendships, etc.

"As hot as it would have been then, given our younger ages and passion, time and energy did not permit us to explore being nonmonogamous.
I have always had what I call the 'sharing' fantasy and desire but kept it
relatively private while our family was so concentrated. When the kids
moved out, there began to be more of a trickle of expressed thoughts and
discussion. Back then we were nearly completely monogamous.

"I had two overnight liaisons with a couple of women that occurred
while I was at professional meetings. I am certain that my wife was scrupu-
lously faithful to me but she certainly got hit on a lot by previous lovers and
other men while at her own meetings and symposia. As our relationship
led up to sharing, I disclosed my previous affairs and she was completely
cool with it—including the previous withholding. She knew that I had very
much less experience than her with such liaisons and didn't mind me having occasional experiences. She's truly an amazing woman! Given the
number of similar affairs she had had, she told me she simply assumed I
would stray occasionally—but that she found her devotion to me nearly
all-consuming.

"The approach to this expansion was perhaps more deepening than the
actual consummation, since we reached another level of disclosing and
discovering fear-related and inhibiting thoughts and feelings. It turned out
that my wife was afraid of losing me, if we explored 'sharing.' She wasn't
afraid so much of losing me to another woman, but afraid of what I would

think of her, if she was with another man, or men. We talked about that a lot, and it deepened our communication, our connection, more than almost anything ever had before. When she had dispelled her fears of losing me with such activities, she told me she thought it would be great to resume more sexual activities. What became apparent to me was that my dear one—as I did—had more or less subsumed a voracious appetite for varied sex in favor of 'marriage.' When we decided to 'expand' our meaning of marriage, there was a definite turning point that brought us closer than ever. Of course the actual consummation was absolutely breathtaking and it turned out we had prepared ourselves very well in the several years it took us to get there . . . time very well spent!

"My wife really doesn't care about the nomenclature of our lifestyle, whether it is cuckolding, or hotwifing, etc. She just knows what she likes and she took to it like a duck to water. We refer to her main lover as our 'house-friend,' a term originally coined by Isaac Singer in a couple of his fabulous short stories about shared wives. This lifestyle is a part of our relationship. We know everything comes to an end and we are prepared for that as much as possible. The principal benefits remain the same: additional motivation to stay in shape, continue exploring the myriad nuances of relationship, excitement, and having a lot of fun. This all feels very natural for us.

"We really don't have any rules left, either. We had our years of a rule-oriented curve, where we set lots of limits about what could and couldn't happen as we explored this. The rules kept diminishing steadily, to where now, we simply acknowledge that she is sexually free to use her own discretion. She is very loving and makes sure that eventually I hear all the details but part of the erotic is that she has her own life. I love it when we get to share together, or when she comes home afterward, and tells me about it while we make love. That is the part of sharing that makes it a fetish for me. There is nothing at all like silky seconds. His presence lingers in her.

"I identify as bisexual especially within a male-female-male threesome (MFM) context. I believe that if we remove the cultural/religious/neurotic trappings, we are all polyerotic. I sometimes do wish my wife were bi, as it would really fill out the dream, but I can be happy with the hand that I'm holding. After all, it's all about our 'attachments' and transitory pleasures. We can't take it with us, so we might as well have the experience to help complete the attachment and then ultimately let go of it and move on. Things seem to work out very well. Love grows.

"My wife is a post-doc scholar and there are few men who can really interact with her at her intellectual level. That said, she loves to be entertained by a good and hard man. She is not so good at just casual small talk, so after the main event, things seem to go downhill. It is a rare thing to find a house-friend who has an intellectual acumen and interest to match hers. Still, we do keep looking and hoping for that right guy who can settle in with us.

"Otherwise we are fairly normal people and this aspect, the sexuality we share with others, does not dominate our lifestyle. It is simply what we enjoy as part of our sexual life. We have varied interests; we love camping, hiking, dancing, playing music together (piano and bass), theater work, travel, family—including my grandchildren, and much more. Perhaps the most unusual aspect of our life is that we don't have a television in our home.

"We have been together for more than twenty-five years now and married for twenty-two. We have been engaged with MFMs for over five years. We were wonderful lovers when first together, and then time, family dynamics, our careers, etc. took their toll on our sexual interest and fascination. We had a tsunami revival upon commencing our particular hotwife lifestyle. It went deep and has affected probably every aspect of our relationship with a big shift in attitude.

"We've moved from automaticity to present and connected communication in all of our endeavors, sexual and otherwise. Before, we lived the way we were expected to live, were told to live, and we made choices, alone and in our relationship, based on those expectations. We were just automatic, like robots. When we started exploring our sexuality together, we started confronting those expectations, those assumptions, and realizing that we could choose other ways, our own ways, ways that involved us being fully present in the moment, in connection with each other. I would like to think that we, with many others, represent a kind of axial shift in how people perceive each other and their ability to create a kind of intentional fusion in any area they choose . . . not without growth and developmental aches and pangs. It's like learning to make music on the instrument of relationship with all the attendant and expected strains and learning curves. Given the general state of the world and the conduct of our nation over the past years, we decided long ago to live a life as much on our terms and desires as possible."

Every couple I met and interviewed offered me surprises, often delightful ones. The philosophical, existential approach that Andrew and his wife brought to their sexual activity was unexpected. I approached this lifestyle believing that what I would find was "extreme sex," equivalent to rampaging, out-of-control sexual behaviors and promiscuity. Instead, what I found, over and over again, were couples who carefully and thoughtfully examined their lives, and chose to act in ways that their free will dictated, rather than what society told them, as it applied to their marriages and sexuality. Some couples that I interviewed actively celebrated their "immoral" and shocking behaviors. Others, like Andrew and Marie, chose to carefully examine their lives, their feelings, their marriages, and their love for each other, and make their own decisions about the role that monogamy should or shouldn't play in their lives.

MONOGAMY AND MARRIAGE

Where did the idea of monogamous marriage first come from, and why? Some anthropologists suggest that marriage and permanent pair bonding serve a valuable, protective role in the history of human evolution and in human society. Without pair bonding, one woman to one man, there may be a constant level of violent, deadly conflict as males fight each other for access to females. Certainly, the origins of polygamy lie in this, with much evidence that polygamy, while common, was prevalent among males who were more economically successful and controlled more power and resources. The emergence of a social orientation towards monogamous dyads reduced intra- and intertribal conflicts, reduced the amount of fighting over women, and may have then increased the degree to which tribes and couples within the tribe could share resources more equitably. With the reduction in time spent fighting over women, tribes could now devote more time to things like farming and hunting cooperatively. Women may have accepted monogamous pair bonding as it reduced the chances of rape and aggression by other males, and increased the security and predictability of food and resources.

In Christian tradition, the tale of Adam and Eve sets the early representation of marriage, with Eve's susceptibility to temptation condemning the couple to be cast out of Eden. Eve is punished with the pangs of childbirth, and is condemned to a subordinate position to her husband. It's not difficult to hypothesize that Eve's susceptibility to temptation had to do with the recognition that women have more sexual capacity than men, and thus may be naturally more susceptible to pleasures of the flesh. The pain (and physical danger) of childbirth might be seen as a warning to women to restrain their boundless sexual capacity.

According to Jewish mythology and tradition, Eve was in fact Adam's second wife. Lilith was allegedly his first wife, created from dust at the same time that Adam was created. However, Lilith was unwilling to lie in the dirt beneath Adam, as they copulated. Instead, she supposedly preferred the position we now term "female superior." Scorning the submissive role, Jewish mythology describes that Lilith was banished, and replaced by Eve. It is likely that Lilith, as a concept, was imported into Jewish tradition, from Mesopotamia, where she was a powerful female demon. In Sumerian and Babylonian tradition, Lilith, sometimes known as Lilitu, was a seductive prostitute of the Goddess Ishtar. She was sometimes referred as a "screeching woman," and came to be associated with the symbol of an owl. In the Book of Isaiah (34:14) the reference to the screech owl that finds rest in Edom may be the only biblical reference to Lilith that remains. Lilith recurs frequently through mythology and literature, including in Goethe's *Faust*, where she is portrayed as an alluring, tempting, but deadly female, who has the power to lead men into danger and death. The icon of Lilith was later incorporated into witchcraft, Satanism, and Wiccan mythologies, where she always plays the role of a powerful, unrepentant, and unashamed female, who consorts with the things man fears and calls evil.

> For on account of a prostitute one is brought down to a loaf of bread, but the wife of another man preys on your precious life. (Proverbs 6:26)

> Such is the way of an adulterous woman; she eateth, and wipeth her mouth, and saith, I have done no wickedness. (Proverbs 30:20)

The Old Testament asserts that female sexuality is a powerful tool, which adulterous women may use at will to manipulate men and acquire what they need. Jezebel was a Phoenician princess who married King Ahab, ruler of ancient Israel. In response to Jezebel's entreaties, Ahab allowed temples to the god Baal to remain in the kingdom of Israel, despite God's commands. Jezebel then used her husband's forces to have the prophets of the Lord killed. Later, Jezebel's husband desired the vineyard of a neighbor, but when the neighbor refused, Ahab merely sulked. Jezebel, disgusted by her husband's weakness, schemed to have the neighbor killed, after having him falsely accused of cursing God and king. For these sins and crimes, Jezebel was at last condemned, thrown out of a window to die, her body consumed by dogs. Although Jezebel's sexuality was never overtly mentioned, her name has come down through history as an epithet for women who use their sexuality to tempt men from the path of God. The term "painted Jezebel" stems from the moments just prior to Jezebel's death, when she takes the time to paint her eyes and arrange her hair, before confronting her accuser.

In Genesis 39, Joseph worked in the home of Potiphar. Potiphar's wife, unnamed in the text, attempts to seduce Joseph, and when he denies her, accuses him of attempted rape. Sentenced to prison for the act, Joseph came to the attention of the Pharaoh and set upon his successful career in government. So, one might argue that Potiphar's wife was doing God's work as she tried to seduce Joseph, in that her lustful, and vindictive, actions led Joseph along the path of his destiny.

Mary, wife of Joseph and Mother of Jesus, "set the bar," so to speak, for the conflict between female sexuality and spirituality in the New Testament. With Christ born to a virgin, conceived by the Holy Spirit, he emerged into the world "untainted" by female sexuality, or sexuality at all. Mary Magdalene, a demon-possessed woman, was saved by Christ, and became one of his closest followers. While not named as a disciple, she figures prominently in all the texts regarding Jesus's ministry. After his death, it was Mary Magdalene who first saw the resurrected Jesus. In a Gnostic gospel not included in the Bible, but found in the Dead Sea Scrolls, the Gospel of Mary Magdalene defends the authority of women to teach the word of Jesus. Mary's relationship with Christ is also explored, particularly the closeness of her relationship with him and the jealousy that other disciples reportedly felt over her intimate relationship with their Lord. While nowhere in the biblical text is Mary Magdalene labeled a prostitute, this label has swirled around her for millennia. In 591, Pope Gregory I gave a sermon where he identified Mary Magdalene as a repentant female sinner, and suggests that her sin was that of adultery. In years to follow, this image gained momentum, such that the image of Mary Magdalene as a woman tainted by sexuality continues to this day.

Early Christian writers such as Tertullian and Augustine argued that even within marriage, sexual intercourse should be reserved for procreation and to prevent "fornication." Chastity was argued for, and promiscuity decried in women. Tertullian urged wives not to tempt their husbands, to control their sexuality, lest it draw men away from the pleasures of the spiritual, into the dangerous depths of the flesh. It was this equation of sex and sin, and particularly with the fear of man's inability to overcome an irresistible female sexuality, that drove the Christian development of celibacy, giving up sexuality for monks, priests, and nuns, in favor of a life in service of God. Sexuality was intended only for procreation, and women were encouraged to suppress any sexual desire or arousal, "submitting" to the husbands' needs. The Jewish tradition of recognizing the wife's needs, and encouraging the husband to fulfill them, was lost in the repudiation of sexuality as sin. Women, as the "receptacle" of sexuality, were also thus tainted.

Some writers have suggested that medieval man in Europe probably did not place much value on or concern about the chastity of his wife, at least, if he was a peasant. Most marriages were economic in nature, without much initial emphasis upon love or even partnership, and often followed directly from a man making overt sexual invitations to a woman. If she accepted, in some cases, the act of sex was viewed as the act of betrothal and marriage. Although Catholic priests and clergy railed against infidelity, and female sexuality in general, their rampant hypocrisy was such that the general populace disregarded it. Clergy were often involved in infidelity and illicit sex, at all levels of the Church. In the fourteenth and fifteenth centuries, various officials within the Catholic Church, from popes to bishops, received taxes and investment returns from brothels, and also sometimes established and covertly managed such establishments.

In the Middle Ages, the idea of "courtly love" began to appear in the arts and literature. It is important to note that in this form, the idea of "pure" love may not have necessarily involved sex (and, according to some, was "purer" when it did not), but did involve the feelings of love between a woman and a man other than her husband. Remember, that in those days, marriages were still arranged, and still about economics and politics. Women were married at very young ages to far older men, who could afford to support a wife and children, and pay the woman's family a dowry. Love could happen, but as in most arranged marriages across cultures, it was a love that was expected to grow from mutual respect, over years of marriage and interdependence, rather than a marriage that grew out of sparks of love.

The Celtic tale of Tristan and Iseult exemplifies this. In this ancient story, dating from as early as 1240, Tristan was sent on a quest to rescue the maiden Iseult, that she might marry his uncle, the king of Cornwall. Successful in his quest, the pair accidentally drank a love potion as they returned to the king's castle. While Iseult does marry the king, she and Tristan continue their love affair until her husband discovers it, and Tristan is forced to flee. This tale is often held up as an inspiration to the tale of the love between Lancelot and Guinevere, with King Arthur as the cuckold.

The most famous medieval love triangle, inspired by the story of Tristan and Iseult, centered on the disastrous relationship between Lancelot, King Arthur, and Queen Guinevere. Said to be the most beautiful woman in the land, Guinevere was abducted, and recovered by Lancelot, Arthur's greatest knight. But, Lancelot and Guinevere fell in love and cuckolded Arthur, in an act that presaged Arthur's ultimate downfall. Arthur himself succumbed to the disastrous sexual wiles of his sister Morgana. But, none of these stories appear in the earliest Welsh tales of Arthur, and they seem to be more elements of high sexual drama, added by Chretien de Troyes, who first popularized much of the tale. Indeed, according to Dante, it was Troyes's story of Guinevere's inflamed passions that led to the character Francesca being condemned to Hell for her adultery, in *Inferno*.

What this tradition of courtly love began to do though, was to foster some acknowledgment of female sexuality. Even married women were encouraged to practice and develop the arts of flirtation, of enticement of men, including their husband. They were especially encouraged to learn to use these arts to enflame passion in their husbands. This cultural swing was not present only in the nobility. Even in the peasantry, songs celebrated the love and passion young wives felt for the young men they chose as their lovers, when their husbands could not satisfy them, as in this song from the Middle Ages:

Fat lot I care, husband, about your love
Now that I have a friend!
He looks handsome and noble
Fat lot I care, husband, about your love
He serves me day and night
That is why I love him so.[1]

However, where Christianity was in ascendancy, sex between man and woman, even husband and wife, was vilified. Sex was endorsed and allowed only for procreative purposes. Men and women were encouraged to avoid any sexual contact not for procreation, and, even in the procreative act, to minimize contact. The "chemise cagoule" was a heavy nightshirt that couples were encouraged to wear during intercourse. Its heavy fabric minimized and deadened any physical contact, and a conveniently placed hole allowed only the necessary physical contact. At this same period, rear-entry sex was prohibited by the Church, not because of its resemblance to animalistic intercourse, but because it was judged to be too stimulating, for both man and woman.

Around this time, even the names of streets began to be changed. In London, a city street (the local brothel district) was long known as Gropecuntlane, but had its name changed, to Grape Street, then Grub Street. Paris had an avenue named *rue Grattecon*, or "Scratchcunt Street." These names were changed in the Victorian era, as open acknowledgment of female sexuality, or sexuality at all, changed. On the Thames River in London, an area now known as Nelson's Dock was once known as Cuckold's Point. The name was bestowed, according to legend, when King John cuckolded a miller, bestowing the land to the wronged husband in recompense. Horns from a stag reportedly marked the spot for many years. In Maine, a stretch of coast that resembled this section of the Thames was named after this London feature. A pair of rocky ledges on the Maine coast were nicknamed the Cuckolds. In Newfoundland, Cuckolds Cove was a site whose name was later changed to Dunfield. Legends suggest the name arose from the story that married women from a nearby fort at St. Johns used this cove for secret assignations. (This cove was later made famous as one of the landing points for the first telegraph lines to cross the Atlantic.)

Thankfully, not all the great, slightly scandalous names were lost to propriety, however. This is especially true in Newfoundland, where residents of the town of Dildo retained their name (they are known as Dildoians). Naked Woman Point, near Trinity Bay on the Avalon Peninsula of Newfoundland, also managed to fend off concerned renamers. Sadly, I was unable to find out the origins of this lovely name—though one can of course presume that there was an unclothed (and probably chilly) woman involved.

Though there is some debate about the precise timing, somewhere around the seventeenth century in Europe and America, marriage began to more closely resemble the marriage of today. Men and women began to seek unions that were based upon love, as opposed to economics. This is not to say though, that marriages were free from strife or contention, now that they were based on love. In 1623, William Whately published an advice book for couples, called *A Bride-Bush or A Wedding Sermon: Compendiously Describing the Duties of Married Persons: By Performing Whereof, Marriage Shall Be to Them a Great Helpe which Now Finde it a Little Hell.* So, that very large section of advice books, on how to turn a difficult marriage into a heavenly one, has a very long historical tradition. I do wonder though, how Whately managed to sell his book without the assistance of television talk shows?

Sexuality within marriage began to return to a level of societal acceptance, with increased cultural norms that supported a mutually rewarding sexual relationship between man and wife. Even as romantic love was growing as the bedrock of a marriage, procreation remained a vital and necessary part of marriage, from society's point of view. Many marriages blessed the union of men and already pregnant brides, as postbetrothal sex became a quietly accepted practice. On the reverse side, impotence, infidelity, and infertility remained acceptable reasons for divorce.

An old saying is "Mama's baby, Papa's maybe," illustrating the fact that maternal lineage is physiologically demonstrable; we know what woman that baby came out of. But paternity? Only today are over-the-counter DNA paternity testing kits available at your local drugstore. Our male ancestors had no effective way to determine if the child they were rearing was really theirs or not. Most studies show that people, including parents, cannot truly tell if a child is related to them by looks alone. People just aren't very good at matching parents to children, by appearance alone. But, when in-laws and relatives see infants for the first time, they often comment upon how much the child looks like the parents. The relatives of the mother tend to comment far more upon the similarities to the father, as opposed to the similarities between baby and mother. In other words, they know that the child is certainly that of the mother, after all it just came out of her body, right?

Given that the child might not be that of the father, the mother's relatives' comments on the baby's similarities to the father serve to protect the child from father's suspicions, by supporting his possibly erroneous belief that the child is his. In the old days, those suspicions might have resulted in infanticide, if the father believed the child was not his, or perhaps in banishment and abandonment of both mother and child. Among primates, many males systematically kill all infants within a troop of monkeys, when they take over dominance of the troop from another male. This assures that they will not invest in the rearing of children of other males, and prompts the females to become sexually receptive to him, as their bodies attempt to create new children to replace those that were slain.

Among the bonobos, known to be extremely sexual, promiscuous, and nonmonogamous primates, hyperpromiscuity by females may be a protective strategy exerted by the females, in order to protect their children from infanticide. Primatologists tell us that when a male primate is reasonably certain a child is not his, infanticide is common. But, in those cases where the certainty is less, and the child *could* be his, a male is less likely to kill the infant, and chance destroying his own genes

Even when the risk is not that of infanticide, there is the risk that men will invest less in their wife's offspring if they suspect the children are not their own. The amount of effort and resources that male swallows allocate to the care of their mates' offspring varies proportionately with how often that mate engages in mating with other males. Studies that used digital morphing technology to create images that were a blend of a human male subject's face and a child showed that the men were more likely to choose these images, over those of other children, when asked if they wanted to adopt a child, or invest resources or money in a given child. Though the men couldn't explain why they chose these children, they could envision sharing their money, homes, and lives, with children that looked like them.

Genetic research over the past decades has indicated relatively high levels of infidelity among modern couples, with some estimates as high as ten percent of births in supposedly monogamous couples actually reflecting extrarelationship sex. One study, reportedly conducted as part of a high school science course, involved testing blood types of children, relating them to parentage. According to the story, a large percentage of the students found that blood testing indicated they were not biologically related to the men raising them. Another investigation, performed with data from the American Association of Blood Banks, revealed that out of nearly three hundred thousand paternity tests, thirty percent of the tests indicated that children had been fathered by outside men.

One Texas man learned that of the four children his wife had borne during their relationship, he was the biological father of only one.[2] The surprised man learned this news after his daughter was diagnosed with a rare genetic disorder, one that children only inherit when both parents carry the genes. Testing of the girl's presumed father revealed he did not carry the gene, and further testing, once the man's suspicions were aroused, revealed that he had fathered only one of their children.

Subsequent studies, using more precise genetic testing to establish parentage, tested children of couples where the males expressed either some suspicion that their child might not actually be their biological child, or where the husbands had no such suspicion. Among those cases where there was suspicion of infidelity, 30–40 percent of the results confirmed the suspicion. Surprisingly, even among those cases where the fathers had no clear suspicion, infidelity was still detected, suggesting that many men may in fact be raising children genetically unrelated to them. Studies in the United States have suggested rates as high as 13–20 percent of children being raised by unrelated fathers, though meta-analytic studies currently suggest U.S. rates are around 4 percent. Similar rates are found in other countries, including Germany (9–17 percent) and Mexico (10–14 percent).

According to the animal kingdom, and research with creatures from insects and fish to birds, apes, and bears, monogamy is exceedingly uncommon in the natural world. In fact, with advances in the technology of genetic testing, many of the species previously lauded as being lifelong monogamous, are now known to actually have many sexual encounters outside their seemingly monogamous partnerships. While they may maintain long-term pair bonds with a single partner, they do not maintain sexual fidelity. Swans, geese, and eagles, species long romantically described as monogamous, have now been revealed to engage in nonmonogamous sexual activity as often as one out of four births. In fact, according to some researchers, it's more newsworthy when evidence of monogamy and sexual fidelity is actually supported in the animal kingdom.

Among mammals, only a very few species live in seemingly monogamous arrangements, and fewer maintain sexual fidelity within those relationships. Man certainly does not seem to be one of them. Rates of infidelity range from 15 to 75 percent, though the most consistent findings suggest that about 25 percent of women admit infidelity across their lifetime, with 40 percent of men acknowledging violations of monogamy within the marriage. These findings may even be low estimates, given the secrecy surrounding extramarital sex.

People commonly make assumptions about infidelity, that the presence of infidelity indicates dissatisfaction within the relationship, at an emotional or physical/sexual level. Pepper Schwartz and Philip Blumenstein argue in their book *American Couples* that these generalized assumptions tend to be unsupported. They describe that there is little difference between couples who are monogamous and those who are not, in terms of the frequency of sex, the satisfaction with sex within their marriage, or even with the level of satisfaction and happiness within a marriage.

A study in Albuquerque, at the University of New Mexico, found that when a husband and wife are too genetically similar, the chances that the wife will cuckold her husband are greatly increased. The similarities between husband and wife were examined in a cluster of genes called the major histocompatibility complex, a clump of genes that appear to be involved in areas of sexual attraction, and immune system response. The more similar the genetics in this complex between a male and female predicts higher feelings of attraction that a female will feel for men other than her spouse or partner, and the greater likelihood that she will have sexual partners outside her primary relationship. Similarity in this area also decreases the degree to which a female responds sexually, with arousal and orgasm, to her partner. According to the study's authors, Christine Garver-Apgar and Steve Gangestad, there was a very strong and reliable mathematical relationship between the genetic similarities and the number of outside lovers that the women reported—if they had half the genes in common, the woman would report, statistically, "half" a lover outside the relationship. Notably, the detection or awareness of this genetic similarity seemed to emerge from a mechanism connected to odor and smell.

When I was in graduate school at the University of New Mexico, they conducted some of these early experiments just down the hall from my office. Female students were asked to sniff t-shirts in plastic bags and rate how attractive they thought the t-shirt's previous male wearer was on the basis of scent. The study revealed connections between attractiveness ratings and the degree of facial symmetry in the males of the study, and later studies suggested relationships between the ratings of attractiveness and genetic similarity in the major histocompatibility complex. Relating these findings to evolutionary theory, they suggest that in a female's quest for improved genetic variability for her children, acquiring genetic contribution from a male with dissimilar genes in this area might improve the immune system response, and overall health, of the woman's child, when compared to genes contributed from a male with similar genes. The similar genes would offer no real change or improvement to the child's immune system.

There was no statistical connection between the degree of genetic similarity in the couple and the male's sexual attraction to his female partner, or to the degree of sexual infidelity on his part. In other words, males don't really care about seeking genetic diversity for their children, and may not even react to the genetic similarity in the way that women seem to. Males, evolutionarily, succeed through seeking quantity, whereas females pursue quality, in the form of genetic diversity, given that their ability to achieve quantity is limited by the number of children their own body can produce. There was also no connection between this genetic similarity, and the degree of marital satisfaction reported by the couple. I find that interesting, given that you would expect some problems, from the increased infidelity and decreased sexual attraction within the couple. However, this offers a reminder that biology is *not* destiny, and that while genes may affect sexual behavior, the love between two people is independent of the drives of their genes.

Biologists examining human sexuality now suspect that male sexuality may have actually evolved in expectation of cuckoldry. The male penis actually works as a semen removal device, with the raised glans (the raised head of the penis) and smaller shaft, where the repeated thrusting of intercourse works to actually scoop out the semen that may be present in the vagina of the woman, increasing the chances of one's own sperm being the one that fertilizes the egg. In a study conducted in 2003 (using various "realistic" sex toys and a semen substitute made from corn starch), researchers showed that the ridge of the glans led to the displacement of 91 percent of the semen already present in the vagina, as opposed to the unridged sex toy, which removed no more than 35 percent of the semen analogue.

In studies with rats, scientists have learned that the number of times the penis is inserted predicts whether or not the female will conceive;

when there are fewer insertions, the female rat is less likely to be fertilized by the male's sperm. Rats' bodies are also somehow able to modulate the amount of sperm they release, adjusting this dependent upon the amount of time that the female has been away from them. The longer she's been away, the more opportunity to be with another male, the more times they thrust and insert their penis, potentially removing more sperm, even as they themselves release more sperm during ejaculation. If another rival male is actually present while the rats copulate, the number of sperm ejaculated by the rat also increases, ostensibly to "combat" the sperm that could be deposited in a moment, by the other male.

When men are jealous, research shows that they tend to thrust longer and deeper during sex, in a manner that would be more effective at removing the sperm of a rival, were it present. So apparently, in group sex encounters in our evolutionary past, it may have actually been adaptive to be last in line, at least for the male.

Not only is the human penis apparently designed to increase reproductive success with promiscuous females, but so are the testicles. Among primate species such as gorillas, where there is little chance that another male has an opportunity to deposit sperm in the vagina of one of the male gorilla's harem, testicles are small. (Although some studies show that fraternal polyandry, when multiple males share a harem of females, is common among as many as 40 percent of some mountain gorilla species; however, the males are always genetically related, and thus, there is less evolutionary pressure upon genetic survival.) There is little need to produce large quantities of sperm to combat the sperm of other males. The testicles of chimpanzees, in contrast, suggest that they evolved in situations where female promiscuity required a great deal of sperm be produced, to outnumber the sperm of other males.

Human testicles seem to fall somewhere in between the average size of chimpanzees and gorillas, and researchers appear split whether this suggests a history of monogamy or promiscuity. Interestingly, some researchers suggest that varying sizes of testicles in individual men sometimes matches behavioral tendencies. In other words, men with larger proportionate testicles may be predisposed to more promiscuous behavior, while men with smaller testicles might be better prepared for monogamy (or life as a cuckold).

Sexual jealousy, at least in males, may have arisen to increase the chances that the child born to a mate was in fact your own. By limiting the chances that she has intercourse with other males, you're limiting the chances that you may raise a child not related to you, and increasing the chances that your genetics and your line of heritability will continue. But, evolutionary biologists suggest that it might have been most adaptive for a woman to choose a "mediocre" male as a primary mate, because such men are better and more reliable caregivers to the woman and her children. More attractive males are more appealing to the woman, but offer less secure nurturance. So, the woman might seek out the more attractive male for illicit sexual liaisons in order to secure for her children the genetic advantages of the attractive male, but remain with her primary mate, who cares for her and her children believing the children are his. Thus, according to this theory, men are in a constant quest to secure the chastity of their wife, to ensure their own genes are passed on, while the wives are in a constant quest to improve the genetic currency provided to their own children, while ensuring those children are raised and cared for.

Montreal social psychologist John Lydon has examined the role of jealousy in married couples. Lydon's research showed that while many married women do experience an initial attraction to other men, those same women very often react to the attraction by working to strengthen and build their relationship with their husband. After meeting an attractive, eligible, and single male in the context of a research study, women were more likely to be forgiving of their husband, generous to his faults. In contrast, married men who met a comparable female in the study were more likely to then judge their wives more negatively, rather than in a forgiving fashion. Similarly, in subsequent related experiments, researchers showed that women were able to mask or control their feelings of attraction towards men other than their husband, able to control or at least limit temptation to flirt. Men were far less able at this skill, having to learn what seemed to come to women naturally.

Monogamy is enforced by law in the United States with criminal adultery statutes, laws against bigamy, and in custody laws. Infidelity is punishable by law in twenty-five states, and is subject to civil lawsuit in eight. While violations of such laws are rarely prosecuted, statutory penalties against these crimes range from two years' imprisonment to commitment for treatment of insanity. Historically, punishment for infidelity in Western cultures has ranged from death to disfigurement. Violation of monogamy by women has typically been punished much more severely than male infidelity. In contrast, other cultures have maintained much less severe punishments against unfaithful wives; in some Inuit tribes, a man whose wife had been unfaithful could challenge the other man to a singing contest, before the tribe. In some tribal cultures, a man whose wife was unfaithful could simply "swap" with the other man, and take his wife. Violation of the expectation of monogamy is a critical component in many modern divorce proceedings, particularly when issues such as alimony and assignment of a couple's assets are considered. Blatant infidelity is the most common reason given for divorce in most cultures across the world. In 1878, the United States Supreme Court ruled that laws prohibiting polygamy were constitutional, and further, that the institution of monogamy was critical to the preservation of democracy.

Infidelity on the part of wives, which presumably became more common as women took on more independent roles outside the home, has remained a reason for divorce. However, old punishments for infidelity have largely vanished, and divorce has become the most common acceptable punishment for infidelity. Across the Western world, laws were passed that now assured that even divorced women could own property and have rights. In contrast to long historical tradition, women were now able to divorce their husbands, though mere adultery was not a sufficient justification. In order to secure a legal divorce, women had to prove their husbands had abandoned them, or were homosexual, perverted, or violent. While the explicit laws governing this may have changed, the implicit social prohibitions behind it remain in place. A study of New Zealand divorce filings shows that while women overall file more frequently for divorce, men who file for divorce citing infidelity by the wife far outnumber the number of divorces sought by wives citing unfaithful husbands.

Even when partners do not sexually violate marriage expectations, with divorce rates as high as 60 percent in some cases, monogamy has less meaning than it once did. Serial monogamy is now the truer term, where individuals are monogamous as long as they are in a given relationship, but move on to other relationships, sexual and otherwise, once that relationship ends. Why then is monogamy the expected, required, and enforced marital ideal? Marriage laws, according to most experts, have more to do with contract and property law. Monogamy offers important assurances regarding parentage that support and clarify inheritance laws and precedents. Some writers and historians suggest that monogamy represents a political and economic compromise, between the needs of the powerful and the need to have a self-sufficient, satisfied, and motivated workforce. Regardless, monogamy works, or at least the idea of monogamous marriage works. A commitment and bond between two partners meets needs for social, emotional, and physical intimacy, as well as financial, familial, and pragmatic needs in ways that no other relationship strategy has as effectively satisfied in current society. But, despite the effectiveness of a seemingly monogamous relationship, history shows that the ideal of monogamy, with the expectation of sexual and emotional fidelity, is not apparently suited for everyone.

An important final point is to highlight an argument made by anthropologist Helen Fisher. Fisher notes that the word monogamy is consistently misused, to apply to a couple maintaining an exclusive sexual relationship, though its original meaning truly applies only to being married to one person at a time. As Fisher says, sexual fidelity between these two people is not a definitional requirement for monogamy. Social and legal discussions of monogamy often equate the two, but sexual fidelity is not a necessary component of monogamy. In other words, it is only arrangements of polygyny or polyandry or group marriage that truly violate the expectation or requirement of monogamy. By definition, so long as a couple remains married only to each other, it doesn't matter who they screw on the side. They may not be maintaining sexual fidelity, but they *are* monogamous. However, for purposes of this book, I will comply with normal, common usage and use sexual fidelity and monogamy as equivalent terms.

BOBBY AND RICHARD

We're just very normal people, but we sure are having fun.

B obby and Richard were the first couple I interviewed in depth. They live in a western city I visited on business and responded to my advertisement on Craigslist. Richard had gray hair, and apologized for dressing casually in slacks and flip-flops. Bobby was slender, with glasses and a meek appearance that disappeared when she laughed. She wore a short skirt that revealed her slim legs, and a silver bracelet on an ankle. Richard is an engineer, with a long and successful career, while Bobby has remained in the home.

They had been married for thirty-six years, were fifty-five and fifty-six years old, and were such an ordinary couple that their lifestyle would be a complete surprise to anyone who knows. It is, in fact, almost as much of a surprise to them. They met in high school, in a small town in a southern state. They were virgins when they started dating and married shortly after graduating high school. Their marriage has been about as middle-class American Dream as it could be. The couple has depended upon Richard's successful career, and Bobby never worked, staying home to raise their four children. The couple has never had serious problems and never considered divorce, or relationship counseling. Neither of them admitted any history of infidelity, and there were no signs that this couple keeps any secrets from each other.

The only hint of stress in their marriage seems to have been around Bobby's role as a stay-at-home mom. While she was home with the children, Richard traveled the world, to spots that Bobby named off with the ease of long recitation. "Brazil, Asia, Europe, Central America, Israel. I went through some hard years. After we had four children, for a few years,

I was depressed. I gained a lot of weight. Some people handle stress by not eating, for me, it was the opposite. Eating was my stress reliever, and I ate, until I was forty pounds overweight."

They sat close to each other during our time together, and communicated with the ease of nearly four decades practice. Both were warm and welcoming, with easy laughs, and were completely candid and forthright. Bobby and Richard had a wonderful communication style, warm, respectful of each other. They clearly had thirty years of experience communicating with each other, and it seems to have been thirty years well spent. They anticipated each other's comments and answers, and there were times when one or the other would pause, as they anticipated their spouse's response. They waited a long time while dating before they began having sex, and both acknowledged they knew little to nothing about sex. According to Bobby, they were both "definitely self-taught in that area."

Richard agreed with his wife. "It's taken years for us to learn. It's been an evolution. We knew absolutely nothing about sex. We grew up in a rural area, around farms, we knew about animal husbandry; saw it every day, so we understood some of the mechanics. But in terms of sex, within a marriage, or especially good sex, we knew nothing."

Bobby spoke up. "Both of my parents were older. My mom didn't even tell me about menstruation. I just had to learn about that on my own one day, much less sex. The only thing she told me about sex was to stay away from it." Bobby laughed again, but there was a slightly bitter quality to this humor, a flavor that hadn't been in her words before.

Richard apparently caught this hint in his wife's voice, and laid his hand on hers. "We weren't in the middle of the Bible Belt, but close to it. It wasn't a subject nice people talked about."

His wife continued. "My girlfriends, we didn't talk about sex. We talked about boys, but not sex. Nobody else knew anything either, so there was really nobody we could learn from, aside from each other."

"We definitely tried to make up for that!" Richard exclaimed. "We had sex a lot, after we were married. Quite a lot of sex, and for a guy, it was satisfying, but it wasn't physically satisfying for Bobby. I imagine it was satisfying emotionally, but Bobby didn't have an orgasm until she was, what?"

Bobby nodded, "I was probably about fifty or so. The kids were older, and I had a talk with Richard one day and said, 'I want to have orgasms, I want to have lots more sex, and by the way, I've never had an orgasm with you in our whole marriage.'"

Bobby's bombshell apparently landed on fertile ground. I can attest to many couples I've seen clinically, where such demands resulted in anger and resentment, even sometimes violence. In many couples, such a statement could not, and often has not been, made by the wife. I was curious how this couple had established such a successful base for their marriage. Given their complete lack of education about sexuality within marriage, where had they learned to communicate so effectively? Richard gave all the credit for this to his wife, describing himself as an "extreme type-A personality," who was pretty hard to live with. Only his wife's patience had, in his eyes, allowed them to have the successful marriage they enjoyed. Bobby was the "peacemaker" in their home, who helped Richard learn to communicate, and to control his temper.

I returned to the topic at hand, with some better understanding of the foundation that Bobby dropped her bombshell onto, and turned to Bobby, asking this slender, meek, peacemaker of a housewife, how exactly it was that at the age of fifty, she went to her husband of thirty years, and demanded more, and better, sex?

"It was partly turning fifty, plus I had eye surgery that left me pretty much blind in one eye. A detached, or torn retina. They had to reattach it, and I don't have much vision in that eye. That and the combination of turning fifty, it took me a long time to adapt. I was home a lot, and had a lot of time to think. You think about getting older, and you want to do things in your life, but now you're on a time schedule, your time is limited. I realized that I wanted to explore my sexuality. I could have orgasms through masturbation, but . . ." her voice trailed off a bit, and her husband stepped in.

"Our sex life was not so hot. It wasn't so much good or bad, but Bobby went into mommy mode, rearing the kids and nesting, and I was interested in work. We just didn't have much sex, and what we had wasn't particularly good. That's a shame, we look back, and we're sad we let that happen. It put some stress on our marriage, but not a lot, surprisingly."

Bobby spoke up in agreement, "We were both busy, tired, stressed. It's hard to keep up the energy for sex, with kids and work and everything. That's partly why we're having so much fun now, because we don't have those demands as much." I saw Bobby squeeze her husband's hand. "Even though our sex life wasn't so good, we always loved each other, very much. And so, well, we had a private moment, in bed together. We talk a lot, together, in bed. Some of our best talks are there, not necessarily having sex, but in bed, talking. And I told Richard . . ."

Richard added, "I was kinda surprised, I gotta tell you. Bobby said, I want to have more sex, and I want to have good sex. Up until then, I think I was convinced she wasn't that interested in sex. Well, I wasn't putting the effort into it I should have, before. And when we did have sex, I felt like she was just doing her duty. So, it was good news to me, but I also felt ashamed, that I hadn't done better on that, over the years."

"I didn't know what fun I was missing," Bobby said, laughing. "In our early years, I explored some, I didn't even know anything, at the beginning, to know I should be exploring. I'm a learner, I read a lot, read everything about sex," Bobby said. "Early on, I started reading those romance novels, I'm sure that was to fill a void. Now, I look back on that, I can see a lot of women make that mistake, thinking it should be that. A lot of women have that idea, that they just have to lay there, and a man should know how to do everything for them. All you have to do is find the right man, the perfect man, and everything will be taken care of. It's taken me a while to get to that point where I knew it was a two-way street, and I knew you don't have to wait for somebody to do it for you, you can take control of it yourself. Now, I've read lots about sex, books on fellatio, books on great sex. Books on multiorgasmic women, because I am one. I'm actually, more than that. I went from none to hyperorgasmic! How?" Bobby shrugged her shoulders. "Don't ask me. It went from orgasms, to, well, it just, I just, exploded. I don't know how it got to that point."

After a moment, Bobby continued, and began to tell about the changes in their marriage, and their sexuality, that resulted from her revelatory demand. "Well, first, it made us close. Richard started buying me sexy underwear, and being more romantic, and I decided to lose the weight I gained, going through that stressful stage. So, I started eating better, walking, going to the gym, and lost forty pounds. That helped in improving our sex life."

Richard nodded, and added, "It also really improved her self-image."

"I had such low self-esteem, I didn't even want to see myself in the mir-ror, much less want to be seen naked. That contributed, and Richard bought me sexy underwear, and we started having romantic times away from home, because we still had kids, in and out of the home. But we had more time alone, getting a hotel, like on an anniversary. Had champagne, strawberries, and we had lots of good sex," Bobby said.

Richard turned to his wife, asking, "How did you have your first orgasm with me? Was it me, putting more effort into it?"

"Probably, I guess," she responded.

Richard turned back to me, saying, "Isn't that a shame, we went for thirty years, without working so hard at it?"

Bobby answered, "Maybe I just showed you what felt good. It's a shame that I didn't do that before."

"But, it was a perfect conjunction. Everything came together, she lost weight, kids were older, she had more free time, and we could travel together."

Bobby added, "We both felt our mortality creeping up on us, and I think we felt, or at least I did, some pressure to live life, in a way that we hadn't before." Bobby and Richard told me how, after a couple of years of "really good sex," they had decided to begin exploring their boundaries. Richard first brought up the topic of swinging, and Bobby eagerly sent her husband on a "reconnaissance mission" to a local swing club. Richard just watched the goings-on at the club, and brought back descriptions to his wife. Both of them were surprised by the quality of people they met in swinging. They had expected to meet "low-class people," and instead, found people like them-selves, who could "think outside the box," and didn't merely accept that life had to be a single way. At first, they didn't have sex with anyone there at the club, but found the environment added to their sexual exploration.

"I thought it was very interesting," Bobby said. "We met people we liked, which was reassuring, and we saw some exciting things. And we would go home, and have hot sex. And then we started talking about do-ing it with another man, having sex with somebody else. There are sites on the Internet, we looked at sites like that together. We found a local, sin-gle man through a site, and we had probably a half-dozen meetings with him, before we decided to play with him.

"Early on, I remember us going on a trip right after getting with Jim, and I remember us lying on the beach, talking about it together. It made our sex really good. After you've done this for a while, what you experience is so much more exciting that anything you see in porn movies, or in erotica. Porn is boring for us now," Bobby smiled.

Richard turned to his wife, "We never watched that much porn, did we?"

Bobby smiled enigmatically, "Not together."

Richard turned back to me and asserted, "Well, I never watched that much porn." Bobby just giggled.

Richard smiled at his wife, and said, "It's easier to find single men. It's harder to find a couple, that you're all compatible with. But, we got with Jim; we were very slow and deliberate. Bobby was very concerned, I think her biggest concern, was how I would feel about her afterwards, if she did have sex with another guy."

Bobby nodded vigorously. "I was worried that he would think badly of me, it might change how he felt for me. Because we've learned that to do this, you have to communicate about everything. You have to let each other know if something does bother you, and so you find yourselves talking about all kinds of things, that. And not just sexual things. That's been one of the biggest attractions to this; after thirty years of marriage, we can finally talk to each other, about anything. Without reservation. It was refreshing. To me, the two big pluses of what we've done, this exploration, is that, and it has been a huge boost to my self-esteem. I never really dated, and I was popular in high school, but since then, thirty-three years, I had only been with him. It just helps you, to know that you're attractive, to a lot of people, not just the one who loves you. It makes a difference. Because you know that your husband, it's more than just a physical thing, with him, as opposed to other men."

Richard expressed a warm, chivalrous sentiment, "A husband does, or at least should, always think his wife is beautiful, no matter what."

Bobby smiled at Richard. "Even if you're really not beautiful. And I think, expressing myself, I've learned. I'm kind of a shy person, but I've gotten out of my shell a lot. And a lot of it is communicating with him, now that's so easy, and now I can express myself with other people better too. That's another thing, I've learned to speak up more."

A more serious look on her face, Bobby said, "I remember going through feeling some guilt, thinking of how people might think of me, if they knew."

Richard agreed, "We both felt that way at first, but that was pretty short-lived too. One of the big changes for me, the culture that we were reared in, the way I was trained, a man was possessive of his wife, and the wife was always subordinate to the male, the husband. And I, to my own credit, had always encouraged Bobby to be more independent." Bobby nodded in agreement, and Richard continued, "And I thought this was a good thing to that end, to help her be more independent."

Bobby added, "That's been one of the big lessons, in that you come to realize that your spouse is not your possession. We love each other tremendously. When we're together, having sex, that's making love. When we're with other people, it's just sex, and it's fun.

"I've never thought really I could end up feeling love for the men I'm with. I feel sexual attraction, but as a friend." Bobby smiled warmly, thinking about the friends she shares her body with. "A genuine affection, I care about them. We do a lot of things with them. Our sex life is really good, alone. We enjoy it tremendously. We're very intimate and close. We have sex a lot, just the two of us. We do it with other men, and that's special too, you can do things with others, that you can't do with just two people." Bobby laughed delightedly. "You can do a lot of different things when you have more than two people. Some couples have different rules from us, about when and where and with whom they can do things. Most of the time, when I go off with other men, Richard isn't there, and that's okay. Part of that is because we've gone through a lot, and a part of that is because I'm very needy for lots of sex," Bobby said this last laughing, and with a tone of pride for her sexual capacity.

Richard nodded, "I have concerns about her safety, but other than that, I don't really have any concerns about her pursuing our hobby without me. When you meet people, you go through an interview process and we've gotten to the point where we can avoid, for the most part, people that we have had problems with in the past. But Bobby is off a lot of times, when I'm not there. I'm gone on work or something."

"He has permission to play with another women, if he wants to, but he doesn't, he's too lazy. It's too much work!" Bobby barked out a short, cheerful laugh.

Richard explained, "For a woman, it's an easy thing to go find guys or couples. I have met women, but it's just a lot of work. I'd rather hang out in my hotel room, and read."

Bobby explained, "I don't do that though, find guys, it's always men that we know, because you want me to be safe. I never go to a hotel bar or something, go off to a room with a guy."

I nodded at Bobby's ankle, balanced delicately on her knee. I'd learned that in the hotwife community, an anklet is sometimes a way that wives advertise sexual availability, and asked if that were the case for them.

Bobby answered, "It's one of the things he got me, along with the sexy underwear. There's kind of a running joke, where people talk online, about ankle bracelets, and some new guy will come onto the forum and say, 'if the woman wears it on one ankle or another, does that mean the woman is a swinger?' They're not really consistent, which is why I'm always switching it up, you have to guess! But really there's no special jewelry or special handshake that identifies strange people like us."

Richard went on, "We have procedures, she calls me before she goes out, and calls me when she gets in and lets me know she's in safe. We've found that we've eliminated rules, as we've gained experience. We've found that when you start in this, you tend to have lots of rules. Some couples, the wife isn't supposed to kiss another guy, that's particularly intimate to them, that's a no-no. Some couples, they can only be in the same room. We have very few rules. As long as no one is getting hurt, and we do try to keep our lifestyle relatively quiet."

"I'm a pretty innocent-looking mom, and we're careful about not being too flagrant about it around the kids," Bobby added. "But our kids did notice a change in us, in me, after we started. I think they like it. It's a positive change."

Richard looked admiringly at his wife. "Confidence is attractive. A really attractive woman, because you see it less in women, is really confident. We've talked to our daughter about that. A really confident woman will walk into a room, and every eye on the room will be on her. She doesn't have to be the most physically beautiful woman in the room. She has that air of confidence. Our kids have said that Bobby is a lot more fun now, more outgoing. We have talked about the possibility of what would happen if the kids find out. We're concerned enough, that we're not flagrant, with our play."

"I worry, I don't want my kids to despise me," Bobby said. "As they get older, it could come to the point where we talk about it maybe, but I wouldn't want it to happen yet, because our daughter is still too young, though, surprisingly, she would probably be the most accepting. Surprising, because she's been the one that's given us the most trouble, she's struggled the most out of our kids. But, because of that, I think she's a lot less judging of others."

Richard said, "We think about getting older, that we will not be as phys-ically attractive, to other people. But on the other hand, we know lots of people in the same boat. They're our age or older, and we figure we'll just age gracefully with our friends. As long as we have an interest in sex, if we want to, we'll do it."

Bobby nodded vigorously. "And when we can't anymore, we'll have lots of great memories. And we won't have that thing, so many people dread, where you regret the things you didn't do. One of the reasons we were willing to meet with you," Bobby nodded at me, "was because we see so much that is the opposite, that people in this lifestyle are bad, so much negative stuff out there. We're not on a campaign to convince peo-ple this is a great lifestyle for everybody, because it wouldn't be for a lot of people. We are just very normal people, but we sure are having fun."

Richard added, "There are lots of ways people do this, some guys get into the cuckold fantasy, where the guy gets enjoyment, watching his wife with another guy. That's not really for us, but Bobby is definitely a *hot wife*! She has hot flashes!" Bobby laughed delightedly. Her husband continued, "For us, it means a wife is a more independent woman, given more lati-tude in expressing and experiencing her sexuality, with herself and with other people."

Richard and Bobby exemplify two of the things I was surprised to find in this lifestyle. First, the amazing degree of communication and mutual re-spect between these two was nothing short of inspiring. As they described, if a couple wants to learn to communicate really well, dealing with the challenges of communication about sexual needs, and sex with others, forces a couple to develop constant, effective, and reciprocal communi-cation techniques. In contrast to the image of dysfunctional relationships participating in swinging, much less the hotwife lifestyle, the relationship between Richard and Bobby was more secure, stable, reciprocal, and mu-tually supportive than many of the "functional" and monogamous rela-tionships out there.

Second, a common concern and reaction to descriptions of the hotwife lifestyle, and to swinging in general, is a criticism based upon feminist principles, and a belief that such choices are male-driven and misogynist in nature. Many people seem to assume that couples participating in this lifestyle do so, only so that the husband can have sex with other women, bartering with other men, using sex with his wife like a commodity. But Bobby was an empowered woman, if ever I've seen one, a woman who embraced her sexuality late in life, and stood up for her own needs. She was lucky to have done so with such a supportive husband, who supported her needs, her independence, his own responsibilities, and yet allowed her the freedom to make her own choices and fulfill her own needs.

Richard and Bobby, late in life, have bloomed into a couple, where Bobby is a wife who is in charge of her own sexuality, and meeting her desire to explore and fulfill her sexuality, with her husband, as well as with other people. But, in contrast to the image of nonmonogamous couples, they proudly proclaim their core "normalcy," embracing this lifestyle as an extension of Bobby's sexuality, and of their mutual desire to explore what life has to offer.

WOMEN, WIVES, AND FEMALE SEXUALITY

Failing to find in women exactly the same kind of sexual emotions as they find in themselves, men have concluded that there are none at all.

Havelock Ellis[1]

"Insatiable." A term that can be used in awe, fear, celebration, and condemnation of female sexual capacity. The Latin root "satietas," means to be sad. The Greek physician Galen wrote that all animals are sad after sex, except for roosters and the human female. The different response of women to sexuality led to the belief that females were somehow vampiric, leeching energy from a man, in the course of sex.

A common myth relating to the fear of female sexual voracity is the myth known as "vagina dentate." This myth, globally present in seemingly independent origins, concerns women whose sexual organs contain teeth that devour the sex of any male so foolish as to penetrate her. A very rare congenital abnormality can in fact create tumorous cysts near the opening of a female's vagina, which could resemble teeth, but the global prevalence of this mythical symbol is believed to have much more to do with humanity's view of, and male's concern with, female sexuality. Legends bearing this element are present in folklore from Europe, Africa, and India, as well as both North and South America.

In the folklore, men combated these toothed vaginas, much as knights fought monsters. In a Jicarilla legend from New Mexico, the boy hero fed the women sour berries that destroyed their teeth, while in a legend from India, the boy hero used an iron tube like an indestructible dildo, to knock out the teeth that lurked in the vagina of a demon female. Catherine Blackledge recounts similar stories in her history of the vagina, asserts that these tales carry similar meaning to that in the Trobiand tale, "pulling vaginal teeth is a metaphor for how some men would like to make women meek and biddable, remolded in a shape defined by them. In these stories, instead of shaming her into submission, physical means are used to tame her sexuality."

Greek mythology describes an argument between Zeus and Hera, over which gender experienced more pleasure from intercourse. They turned to Tereisias, a man who had been punished by the gods to live as a woman for seven years. Notably, when living as a woman, Tereisias was a bit promiscuous, and a very popular prostitute. Tereisias answered that, "If the sum of love's pleasure adds up to ten, nine parts go to women, only one to men."[2] The founder of the Muslim sect of Shiites said something very similar, that nine parts of sexual pleasure were given to women, and only the remaining one was for men. In Hindu legend, a king who angered the gods was transformed into a woman. When at last forgiven, the king was offered the chance to return to manhood. Based upon the greater pleasure felt as a woman, the king chose to remain a queen, or, at least, a woman. An ancient aphorism, sometimes attributed to Muslim tradition, and other times to the Old Testament, suggests in the world, there are three things that are insatiable, the earth (or the desert), the grave (or Hell), and the female vulva.

Witch hunts, conducted throughout Europe and America from the fifteenth to the eighteenth centuries, focused primarily upon women. The hunts began nearly four hundred years before, in efforts to rid Europe of heretics. But, in 1487, the publication of the *Hexenhammer*, also called the *Malleus Maleficarum*, known as the Witch-hunter's Bible, gave explicit directions for identifying and capturing witches who used Satan's power in an affront against God and the Church. The Witch-hunter's Bible asserted that the female insatiability for sexual pleasure was the way in which the devil gained power over women, also reported that many of these witches could either steal a man's penis, or make it disappear. The witches could also impose sterility upon a male enemy, by preventing the flow of semen, through use of their magic and curses. When the witches stole penises, they seemed to have sometimes kept them like pets, shutting them up in boxes, and feeding them "oats and corn." (Nice of them; they could have just let the poor things starve.)

Female capacity for sexual pleasure was specifically cited in the *Malleus Maleficarum*. Women are "more carnal than a man," and "the word woman is used to mean the lust of the flesh." Indeed, "All witchcraft comes from carnal lust, which is in women insatiable," given as a reason for female vulnerability to Satan and to the powers of witchcraft.[3] As in the story of Eve, the greater female capacity for sexual pleasure equates to a greater temptation to its power.

It is this insatiability that, according to some sociologists and anthropologists, led to the suppression of female sexuality in human history. The argument led thus, that unless female sexuality was suppressed, confined, and restricted, human society would be a sexually driven chaos. (A corollary of this argument is used to explain a possible evolutionary purpose of the female orgasm. Females who were more orgasmic were more likely to have sex, and thus more likely to reproduce, and their descendants would thus outnumber the descendants of females who did not have orgasms). Apparently, if human females indulged their sexual appetites, the endless orgies might have gotten in the way of the invention of the wheel, discovery of fire, and so forth. Oh, and the men would have to take care of the kids, because the moms would be too busy, umm, getting busy.

Mark Twain humorously described the mismatch between the sexual capacity of females, and the male ability to satisfy this capacity, suggesting that this paradox was reflective of God's sense of humor, and man's irrationality:

Now there you have a sample of man's "reasoning powers," as he calls them. He observes certain facts. For instance, that in all his life he never sees the day that he can satisfy one woman; also, that no woman ever sees the day that she can't overwork, and defeat, and put out of commission any ten masculine plants that can be put to bed to her. He puts those strikingly suggestive and luminous facts together, and from them draws this astonishing conclusion: The Creator intended the woman to be restricted to one man.

So he concretes that singular conclusion into law, for good and all.

And he does it without consulting the woman, although she has a thousand times more at stake in the matter than he has. His procreative competency is limited to an average of a hundred exercises per year for fifty years, hers is good for three thousand a year for that whole time—and as many years longer as she may live. Thus his life interest in the matter is five thousand refreshments, while hers is a hundred and fifty thousand; yet instead of fairly and honorably leaving the making of the law to the person who has an overwhelming interest at stake in it, this immeasurable hog, who has nothing at stake in it worth considering, makes it himself!

You have heretofore found out, by my teachings, that man is a fool; you are now aware that woman is a damned fool.

Now if you or any other really intelligent person were arranging the fairness and justices between man and woman, you would give the man one-fiftieth interest in one woman, and the woman a harem.[4]

Another possible motivation for social suppression of female sexuality, explored by psychologist Roy Baumeister and colleague Jean Twenge, was that males might be, at core, simply jealous of female sexual capacity. Baumeister and Twenge argued that there is little evidence that male jealousy is a significant factor in the suppression of female sexuality. They suggest that in fact, men tend to be eager and responsive to the opportunity, to any opportunity, to satisfy a woman sexually. In many surveys, men as a whole come across as less selfish than women, sexually, reporting that giving a partner sexual pleasure is more important than their own.

Research studies have shown that most men will respond affirmatively and eagerly to unknown women who make sexual requests, whereas women are less responsive to spontaneous sexual offers from strange men (all over the world, women read this research and are less than surprised). A woman's perceived or real promiscuity greatly increases the degree to which males find her attractive. Men simply appear to be programmed to respond with lust towards those women they perceive as available, as the lusty response motivates the male's pursuit of a reproductive opportunity. Evolution rewarded the genes of men who responded to every woman who seemed to be available. In contrast to many other mammal species, human females show no overt signs of fertility or ovulation, and are capable of sexual response throughout their ovulation cycles. Some studies have indicated that single women are more likely to wear revealing clothing when going out "clubbing" around their ovulation, and this is an easy signal to mimic. In other words, females may choose to be sexually provocative and inviting even when not ovulating, and "fool" men into mating with them, providing the woman with sexual pleasure. Men may be programmed to submit to such fooling, in order to seize every opportunity in which they might pass on their genes. Mae West famously described this effect, and said: "Men like women with a past because they hope history will repeat itself."[5]

On the website OurHotwives.org, men and women celebrate, discuss, and argue the nature of their sexual lifestyle. One husband described how he first discovered his wife's sexual promiscuity and infidelity when, three months after their wedding, she was dropped off at his home, late one night, by two black men. His wife's clothes were disarranged, stained with semen, and her neck covered with bite marks. Aroused beyond his belief, the man and his wife had sex all night. His wife disclosed the extent of her infidelity to him, as well as a true account of her sexual history, involving many more men than he ever knew. The husband then kept a diary of sorts, recording his wife's sexual encounters with other men, over the course of their twenty-five year marriage. He stated, emphatically and precisely, that his wife had been with 372 different men throughout their marriage, including nine men in a one week period, and seventeen different men during the course of a weekend "stag" party, where she was the entertainment.[6]

The most well-supported argument to explain the history of the suppression of female sexuality, according to Baumeister and Twenge, is that men might not be the main culprits, but women. Using an argument developed from social exchange theory, a model of social interactions that is based upon economic principles, they argue that women have historically had little to offer, aside from their sexuality. As a result, in order to keep the "price" of sexuality high, and the value stable and dependable, women had to control the "market" for female sexuality. When I talked about this with my wife, she commented on what her grandmother had told her: "No one's going to buy the cow, when they can have the milk for free." (Sexual advice columnists in women's magazines often tell women readers that when they want a "real" relationship, they should withhold sex, until they know how the man really feels about them. "Play hard to get.")

So, because sexuality was, historically, one of the only "valuable commodities" men wanted, and women controlled, females began to punish women who drove down the price. British journalist Lynn Barber, a former writer for *Penthouse*, described her childhood.[7] As a girl, she was taught that girls hate sex, yet she found herself growing fascinated and intrigued with girls who had sex. Lynn describes that girls were taught that sex should be expensive, and should cost males an expensive fee in dinner, entertainment, and attention. Lynn points out nicely that she and other girls were trained to treat their sexuality as a commodity, much like any prostitute. Only sluts had sex for free.

Programs funded to provide abstinence-only education explicitly support this message, with curricula that direct females to be conscious that their dress and appearance might inspire "lustful thoughts" in males, a situations that girls are responsible for avoiding. Abstinence-only curricula go on to support the notion that females have no interest in sex outside a relationship, unless they are using the sex to meet needs for attention or "insecurity."[8]

It is fascinating, however, that when women are coached by advice columnists on how to "spice up" their relationships, and "fire up" their husbands, they are usually told to engage in behaviors that would be labeled as slutty in other circumstances—wearing revealing clothes, initiating sex in "risky situations" like in the movie theater or at the office. Michele Weiner Davis, author of *The Sex-Starved Wife*, offers many of these tips, including:

> Tell him you're not wearing panties. Whispering this to him in public is especially good. Wear a blouse or shirt that hangs open when you bend over, and flash him.[9]

An important caveat here is to point out the core truth that sexuality "costs" females more. The risks of becoming pregnant, the medical risks of pregnancy itself, the risk of having to potentially rear a child are all dramatic, expensive potential "costs" that men do not risk to the degree that women do. Thus, it makes sense, from the economic argument, for women to guard sexuality more carefully than men—the female ratio of returns versus risk for sexuality is far lower than men, even considering the greater orgasmic and sexual capacity in females.

The "principle of least interest" is an economic concept suggesting that the person least interested in the desired outcome often has the greatest control of the price. The person haggling with you over the price of the apple at your fruit stand is apt to get a better price out of you, if they seem like they'd be just as happy to eat gravel than your apple, and they're only bargaining for the heck of it. In Latin American markets, I always get the best deal when I start to walk away, and act as though I've given up. So, women who have convinced men that sexuality is just not all that interesting or rewarding for the woman have a lot more control over how much the man is going to have to invest, in order to get sex "from" the woman.

Following from these arguments, those outlets where men can get sexual stimulation more cheaply would hurt "the market," and thus be a problem for women. Historically, it has been women and female-driven lobbies that oppose, prohibit, and limit such things as prostitution and pornography, again, as those outlets are "cheaper" than the going rate that women need. (Indeed, research on prosecution of prostitution shows overwhelmingly that it is the prostitute who receives the greatest punishment—the "johns" are often simply released with no charges, or with charges that are far more minor than those experienced by the female prostitutes.) Baumeister and Twenge say it clearly:

> Women benefit economically if men are starved for sex, whereas men benefit sexually if women are desperate for money and other resources.[10]

Substantial research has shown that women who are more independent financially, more educated, and less dependent upon their husbands are rather more likely to have sexual affairs, and also more likely to enjoy sex and pursue it for their own pleasure.

Research with females and sexuality offers numerous examples, many gathered by Baumeister and Twenge, showing the degree to which females suppress and limit the sexuality of other females (note, this isn't judged as a bad thing, but just the way it is—often, in the examples below, there are real risks these females are trying to protect other women from):

- When males go on spring break, they often agree to help each other "get laid." When women go on spring break, they much more often set up arrangements to get each other out of sexual situations and prevent each other from going "too far."
- The degree of close communication between mother and daughter predicts the daughters' sexual activity—the more communication,

the less the daughter is sexually active. Degree of communication with father has no impact on the daughters' sexual activity.

- In female friendships, the sexual activity level of one friend tends to be consistent with the rate of the other female. Contrary to many assumptions, when a girl begins to have sexual activity or loses her virginity, they don't usually "drop" their friends that aren't having sex, taking up with girls who are. This is because once one girl begins to have sex, it increases the likelihood that her friends will soon follow.
- In high school, it is girls who condemn and shun other girls for sexual activity.
- The "double standard," that some sexual activities are okay for males, but not females, is far more supported by women than men.
- Gossip by other women, and the reputation one holds among other women, are often cited as the most powerful influences on women to "hold back sexually."
- Highly sexual women (those who report wanting sex at least seven times a week or more) report that they typically have much better relationships with men, including just friendship, and relatively poor friendships with women. Men are more accepting of these highly sexual women, and far less judgmental.

In the early 1900s, British sex researcher Havelock Ellis wrote: "Before sexual union the male tends to be more ardent; after sexual union it is the female who tends to be the more ardent. The sexual energy of women, under these circumstances, would seem to be the greater on account of the long period during which it has been dormant."[11]

As the politics of the world began to change, with increasing democracy and freedom of speech sweeping across America and Europe, so too did the role of women and wives. Wives (though not necessarily single women) began to be increasingly represented in political, scientific, and philosophical discourse. Though single women involved in such activities were still perceived as aggressive and unladylike, wives who did so were accepted, so long as their activities supported their husbands. The earliest feminist writers, such as Mary Wollstonecraft, began to publish their works, calling for greater freedom for women.

In the late eighteenth and early nineteenth centuries, Victorian scientists demonstrated that female orgasm was not necessary for conception. As this discovery spread, the notion of female sexuality was turned upside down, from woman as insatiable temptress to woman as physically cold, sexless, and merely capitulating to the greater sexual drives of their husbands. Writers of the time believed that women were untroubled by sexual desires.

Historically, female sexuality was seen as the core cause of most problems in females. The term hysteria, typically applied predominately to women, originated from the concept that unfulfilled female sexuality was unhealthy. In Greece, female hysteria was attributed to a "wandering uterus," which was dry and went wandering in the body for moisture, ending up in the throat and chest, choking the woman. Plato suggested that the uterus was so "hungry" for procreation, and reproduction, that when unsatisfied, it wandered through the body to create havoc that ultimately forced the woman to seek sexual contact. Likewise, Freud suggested that the female's uterus, and need for procreation and reproduction, drove her personality development, leaving it, and her sexual fulfillment, dependent upon the male penis, and male power. Along with the vulvular massage techniques, physicians also used scented and aromatic oils, along with recommendations for horseback riding and rocking in swings and hammocks. Although these treatments appear unbelievably naive and blind to us, not all physicians were unaware of the orgasmic results of their actions. Some described their treatment as initiating orgasms, or something similar. While abuses no doubt did occur, with physicians taking advantage of their female patients (some records suggest that the most likely to be thus treated were young widows), most of these doctors believed in the benefits of their actions.

In the 1880s, Kelsey Stinner invented an electrically powered vibrating device that was embraced by physicians as a labor-saving tool in their provision of "vulvular stimulation" to countless "hysterical" wives. Doctors had, for many years, treated female hysteria, otherwise known as genital congestion, with a manual pelvic massage that eventually resulted in a "hysteric paroxysm" that ultimately relieved the woman of symptoms such as shortness of breath, fainting, and, I'm not making this up, "troublemaking." Of course, such release of symptoms was a temporary fix at best, and women would return often for treatment. These doctors struggled with the physical fatigue of their altruistic labors, and complained of the time and effort it required of them. To save their strength, alternatives were introduced, from "hydrotherapeutic devices" that resembled today's Jacuzzi jets to steam- and clockwork-powered vibrating machinery (the steam-powered "Manipulator" was introduced to great fanfare in 1870s London). As the convenience of electric power was tapped, these vibrating devices spread from the doctor's office, to the pages of even the Sears, Roebuck catalog and ladies' magazines, where they promised to promote health, beauty, and life. A visit to the Good Vibrations Store, a feminist cooperatively owned sex toy store in San Francisco, allows one to view a glass-encased display of vibrating devices from this period.

Over the past few years, vibrators have become the subject of much legal attention, as the states of Alabama and Texas have attempted to prevent their sale. For nearly a decade, Alabama has tried to press laws against the sale of such devices within state lines. Federal appeals courts have supported Alabama's stance, and, according to sexologist Marty Klein, have "ruled that the government has a compelling interest in keeping 'orgasm stimulating paraphernalia' out of our hands."[12] The day appears to be returning, when, at least in some states, a doctor's involvement may again be necessary for a woman to use a vibrator to gain an orgasm.

And yet, even as labor-saving tools were devised and implemented, to save doctors the strain of inducing orgasms in housewives, day after day, there remained a core medical belief that the majority of women were not very troubled with sexual feelings. The view was occasionally challenged, as it was by Dr. Elizabeth Blackwell in 1894. The first female doctor in the United States, she argued that distinguishing male and female sexuality was futile, and posed significant social risk, as women were denied access to expression of sexuality. The late 1800s were also the times of Dr. John Harvey Kellogg, who championed the fight against the ills of masturbation, and drastic, sometimes horrific, treatments to prevent masturbation. Whereas prior, the "retention of seed" (in both males and females) had been condemned as resulting in madness and illness, masturbation was now condemned as destructive to a woman's sexuality, decreasing her ability to experience or even feel sexual pleasure.

Led by Freud, thinkers of the nineteenth and early twentieth centuries saw female sexuality as subservient to male sexuality, and clitoral orgasm was immature and inferior to the vaginal orgasm, an orgasm triggered by the penetration of the penis. Clitoral orgasms, and orgasms that resulted from masturbation (typically emerging from clitoral stimulation), and even orgasms that resulted from the "female superior" position, with the woman on top of the man, were decried as immature, inferior, and evidence of poor or incomplete personality development in a woman.

When Western society was working to deny the capacity of female sexuality, and to redefine women as "pure" and less sexual, those women who exhibited obvious, overt sexuality stood out from the crowd. When women were acknowledged as, at core, sexually insatiable by virtue of their femininity, sexually voracious women were sometimes celebrated as simply being very female. Such women were indeed celebrated as temple prostitutes and priestesses, when sexuality was regarded as sacred. But, when the idea of woman was redefined, to be less sexual than men, these women, and their sexual desires, became pathological, and evidence of a disease. Such women were labeled as nymphomaniacs, their pathological sexual desires blamed on mental illness, overly large clitorises, masturbation, poor diets, and other physical maladies. Because women were viewed as less sexually capable than men, some episodes of nymphomania were believed to be caused by the psychological "scarring" of a woman's brain, when she was exposed to sexuality or sexual incidents that were so powerful they "overloaded" that poor woman's brain and somehow supercharged her libido, beyond her ability to restrain it. In contrast, in 1775, medicine identified that masturbation was the chief cause of nymphomania, and the inability of a woman to control her sexual desires, succumbing to overwhelming sexual excess and indulgence.

Nymphomania was "treated" with everything from medications, psychotherapy, surgery, electric shock, and removal or excision of the clitoris, at least, that part of it, the glans, which could be "easily" removed. Thus, many women who had their clitoris surgically removed continued to have sexual response, and orgasm. Because these women believed, as their families and doctors told them, that their sexual response was evidence of illness, their continued experience of arousal and orgasm was seen as a problem, and a measure of the insidiousness and power of this illness.

Not all women readily went along with or accepted the limitations put upon them, and their sexuality, by the "experts." In her delightful book

Nymphomania, A History, Carol Groneman recounts the tale of a twenty-five-year-old woman, who complained that doctors had "de-sexed" her after she was hospitalized and treated for being a "psychopathic nymphomaniac."[13] The woman was reputed by the doctors to collect men like postage stamps, and even supposedly "cohabitated" with ten members of a football team in one night, though, sadly, the players supposedly lost their game on the day following this woman's affections. This last detail was almost surely thrown in by the doctors in order to support the notion of female sexuality as a form of vampirism, or merely as a throwback to the belief that retention of a male's "seed" improved athletic and combat performance. But, after being released from the hospital, this woman returned to her former ways, unrestrained by the doctor's treatments.

Alfred Kinsey was one of the most famous and influential sexuality researchers, opening the doors of sexual exploration, throughout American bedrooms, including his own. An entomologist originally, Kinsey also had strong interest in sexuality, both personally and professionally. As described in biographies, Kinsey had a history of exhibitionism and nudism, even prior to developing interest in sexology. Stories by graduate students describe long conversations with Kinsey around their sexual experiences and masturbatory habits, conversations in which Kinsey openly shared his personal experiences.

Sexual research conducted by Alfred Kinsey led to explorations of sexuality by both he and his wife, Mac. Biographers such as James Jones report that Kinsey explored both his own homosexual urges, and masochistic and exhibitionist urges, as his career progressed. Kinsey allowed, and indeed encouraged, a free sexual environment of exploration among the team of researchers he gathered around him. Kinsey reportedly decreed that within his circle of researchers and friends, sexual liberation was to reign, with male homosexuality allowed, and that wives could be shared with each other. Wives as well were free to choose and pursue their own sexual explorations; Kinsey's sexual utopia was not a chauvinistic one. He extended sexual freedom and choice to women, as well as men. When marital infidelity was involved though, Kinsey required that he be consulted, in order to determine whether such a relationship was to be permitted or allowed.

It was with apparent sadness that Kinsey directed an employee to cease his sexual relations with another researcher's wife, due to the negative impact the relationship was having on the other researcher's marriage. No such impact was apparently evident as Kinsey readily shared his wife Mac with numerous other men. Multiple researchers, and family friends, describe having sex with Kinsey's wife, sometimes with Kinsey there and participating, other times alone with Mac. When Clyde Martin, a student and sometime male lover of Kinsey, asked Kinsey if he could approach Mac for sex, Kinsey reportedly responded that he hadn't thought of this, but had no qualms or reservations. Indeed, at Kinsey's encouragement, his forty-two-year-old wife was tasked with "educating" young Clyde in sexual encounters with women, ostensibly passing on the sexual repertoire that she and Kinsey had acquired through their own explorations. It is considered possible, by Kinsey's biographers, that some of Kinsey's willingness to share his wife sexually emerged from Kinsey's sexual attraction to males, and to Clyde particularly.

Some of Mac's sexual encounters with others were filmed, in a private studio in Kinsey's attic, where Kinsey orchestrated filming of sexual encounters by numerous volunteers and fellow researchers. Some sessions involved filming of masturbation, by Mac, and others (including Kinsey himself); others involved filming of sexual encounters, between both hetero- and homosexual couples, as well as group sexual encounters at Kinsey's direction. Few films reportedly included Kinsey himself, possibly due to his supposed difficulties with erectile dysfunction, likely due to physiological problems. (One of the male insiders from Kinsey's circle later suggested that this physiological difficulty might have also contributed to Kinsey's arrangement of sexual partners for his wife, unable to physically meet her needs.) Even those sexual encounters in the attic that didn't include Mac in the action, as it were, often included her involvement as she brought refreshments to the participants, as hostess, and perhaps as another effort to include herself in her husband's work.

In his text reporting the results of sexual interviews with females, Kinsey appears to have struggled with his personal and professional conceptualization of female sexuality. He clearly maintained the Victorian notion that female sexuality was less than that of male sexuality. In his research procedures, he acknowledged that research with female sexuality was inhibited by the social pressures against full female disclosure, and made effort to accommodate for this in research and interview procedures. Kinsey clearly had notions and intent toward social change, with regards to sexual liberation. His view of female sexuality as "less" was in contrast to this, a view that Kinsey made effort to change in his writing and research. However, despite females who reported great sexual capacity and desire, Kinsey retained a view of female sexuality that was inhibited compared to male sexuality. Kinsey identified that women in his sample had fewer orgasms and sexual interests than men, both before and after marriage. Many women reported a complete lack of orgasm, despite long marriages and sexual relationships.

As with male sexuality, Kinsey reported extensively on female involvement in extramarital sex. He identified that many women, as well as men, engaged in sex outside their marriage. According to Kinsey, many of the described extramarital encounters had few, if any, negative consequences. Kinsey did describe that infidelity could and did cause conflict and problems, but stated that such results were avoidable. He reported that some women engaged in sexual encounters outside their marriage, due to boredom, sexual dissatisfaction, and intense friendships, as well as love affairs. Extramarital sex, as reported by wives, sometimes even improved and enhanced the sexual relationship within the marriage. Kinsey suggested that unless both marital partners were equally "strong-minded," extramarital sex was best kept secret, to preserve a relationship.

Kinsey conducted interviews with couples, presumably where both partners were in fact "strong-minded," where wives had sex outside their marriage, with full consent and knowledge of the husband. Kinsey described that while some men did encourage their wives into extramarital sex, so that the men could pursue their own extramarital (sometimes homosexual) activities, many of the men did so in an honest attempt to give their wives the chance for sexual fulfillment. Kinsey's biographer Jones quotes passages from Kinsey's description and explanations of permissive female extramarital sex, and suggests that Kinsey was being especially self-referential, using the data to explain his own predilections for sharing his wife Mac with other men.[14]

Thus, Kinsey's explanation of wife sharing reflects many of his own apparent motivations: altruistic desire for his wife to experience sexual satisfaction, beyond and in spite of his own limitations; support and implicit permission for his own extramarital sexual encounters, primarily with other men; and opportunity for Kinsey to explore his homosexual inclinations through voyeurism and direct action with the men with whom he shared his wife. Kinsey's arguments nicely foreshadow my own, suggesting that the search for a single explanation for wife sharing is fruitless. Even in a single couple such as the Kinseys, there were multiple causes which supported Alfred's sharing of his wife's sexuality with other men.

At the same time as the revolution brought on by Kinsey's works, female authors such as Marie Bonaparte wrote that women were endowed with less libido, and were less able to fulfill their sexuality than men. It is worth noting that Marie Bonaparte was a protégé of Freud, and had sought treatment from him for her inability to experience orgasm in missionary position. Deciding on her own, and based upon physiological research that she herself conducted, that the cause was the distance between her vagina and clitoris, Bonaparte had her clitoris removed surgically, and an attempt was made to graft it closer to her vagina. The attempt failed to improve her sexual response.

One reason that the attempt failed is that the anatomy of the clitoris is far from the "tip of the iceberg" that can be seen. In 1561, the Italian scientist Gabriel Fallopio (one of the first inventors of the condom, though his fabric sheath was less comfortable than the intestine condom later popularized by Conton) identified that the structures of the clitoris extend far deeper that previously realized. In 1672, a Dutch anatomist argued that there were core flaws in the analogy that the female clitoris was the homologue of the male penis. Even the ancient Greek physician Galen argued that the vagina was the equivalent of the penis, "turned inside out," and the clitoris played an integral anatomic role. As previously described, many of the women who experience clitorectomies, or culturally driven surgical excisions of the clitoris, are still able to experience orgasm, though they go to pains to conceal this fact from their husbands. The clitoris is merely the tip of a larger anatomical structure in the female sexual organs. But, this knowledge was mysteriously "lost" to medicine and science, and was only rediscovered by Western society in the latter half of the twentieth century. It is speculated that this loss of knowledge may have been related to the seventeenth-century view of the clitoris as the "seat of sin," because it was also the primary seat of female sexual pleasure. The great sensitivity and responsiveness of the clitoris was related to, and perhaps even responsible for, the female susceptibility to evil, as detailed in the Witch-hunter's Bible. So, by denying clitoral pleasure, "Victorian men made their wives pure, nearly virginal, and faithful—or so they hoped."[15]

In the 1960s, sexuality researchers William Masters and Virginia Johnson began pioneering research in St. Louis, Missouri, picking up where Kinsey left off. After interviewing many prostitutes about the mechanics of sexual behavior, they then moved on beyond mere interviews. Recruiting male and female participants, they measured, analyzed, and recorded the physiological components of sexual arousal, sexual intercourse, and orgasm. Their research supported the need for clitoral stimulation for female orgasm, but further, empirically documented, for the first time, a core difference between male and female sexual response. According to Masters and Johnson's research, males, following orgasm, demonstrate a refractory period, in which they are physically unable to achieve another erection or orgasm. Females show no such limitations. As Sherfey went on to show, female sexuality, at a physiological level was capable of, perhaps even made for, greater sexual capacity then male, with increasing orgasmic response as sexual stimulation continued. She viewed female sexual response as innately insatiable, celebrating this boundless capacity in contrast to the long millennia of fear and rejection of female sexual capacity. Following the surge of Masters and Johnson's research and therapeutic methodologies, it was now male sexual inadequacies that came to the forefront. Male impotence, premature ejaculation, and inability to provide their female partners with satisfactory orgasms and sexual experiences now generated tremendous attention. Whereas before, female sexuality was viewed as less than that of males, the turning of the coin now put tremendous pressure upon males across America, as women began to assert their sexual needs in the bedroom.

Masters and Johnson also attacked the long-held belief that women do not respond to pornography. Though women reported subjectively little arousal, the researchers used physiological data revealing blood flow and lubrication in the vagina to show that women responded physically, and almost instantly, to sexual imagery. This research has continued over the years, and shows even further that women's physiological sexual response is almost "pansexual" when compared to males. Heterosexual males respond to heterosexual pornography, but their penises show little response to male homosexual imagery. (The exception is males who report high levels of antihomosexual beliefs. These guys do typically respond with a homosexual arousal pattern. Sweet irony.)

But women, regardless of their identified sexual orientation, demonstrate physiological arousal to sexual imagery, whether it is hetero-, homo-, or bisexual. One study conducted in Toronto by Meredith Chivers showed that women even responded with physical arousal to film of bonobo monkeys mating, while males showed no such response. Chivers has described how female sexuality is more "receptive" and "reactive," despite female sexuality being greater than that of males. University of Nevada psychologist Marta Meana has similarly suggested that female sexuality is somewhat more "narcissistic" than male sexuality, based upon a core female desire to be sexually desired.[16]

Thanks to research by Masters and Johnson, the clitoris, the clitoral orgasm, and the multiorgasmic female, all began to be at least socially acknowledged as normative, if not fully embraced as healthy. They argued that labels and diagnoses of nymphomania emerged from the lack of understanding of female sexual response, and particularly of the female multiorgasmic capacity. But, the mental health field was unwilling to just toss away such a useful concept as nymphomania. So, clinicians applied yet another moral judgment and assumption. Following the revolution brought on by Kinsey and Masters and Johnson, women who were merely highly sexual could no longer be effectively labeled as pathological. But, women who had sex with men that they did not love, women who engaged in group sex or anonymous sex, women who were promiscuous, and did not "settle down and fall in love," were clearly pathological.

The idea that only men enjoy sex outside love was the core assumption of the reconception of pathological female sexuality, which led to women, and particularly, female teenagers, committed to psychiatric hospitals and treatment centers for the "illness" of promiscuity outside marriage or even a loving relationship. It was rare then, and still is, for a male teen, even a homosexual male teen, to be similarly forced into treatment by courts, physicians, and families for the sin of promiscuity. The most common justification for these forced treatments, which still go on today, is that by virtue of her promiscuity, the teenage girl is placing herself at physical risk of disease and pregnancy.

The wave of sexual revolution crested in the 1960s, with the availability of the female contraceptive pill. (Although approved by the FDA in 1960, the American Medical Association opposed contraception until 1965. The overwhelming majority of doctors had no training in sexuality or contraception, and often vigorously opposed efforts to liberalize society's sexual morals and practices.) Across generations of females, women began to embrace and express their own sexuality, asserting their own control over their bodies, their pleasure and arousal.

As women as a group began to acknowledge a desire for sexual pleasure, without the requirements of love, monogamy, and commitment, and were safe from pregnancy in their pursuits, the definition of pathological female sexuality shifted yet again. (The assumption that women can only achieve real sexual fulfillment in loving, caring, and romantic relationships remains a common theme, found in clinical works, as well as popular women's magazines, which drive home the frequent message that for a woman, sex with someone you love is better—a subjective assessment more loaded with moral judgment than empirical backing.)

Nymphomaniacs were now recast as sexual compulsives, who pursued their anonymous, degrading sexual encounters out of a deep-seated sense of internal loathing. By masochistically seeking out men and sexual encounters that were unhealthy, dangerous, and that involved little sense of respect for the woman's sexuality, so the theory went, the woman found external confirmation of the feelings of emptiness inside. Other theories, still present in the current version of the American Psychiatric Association's *Diagnostic and Statistical Manual of Mental Disorders*, linked unhealthy female promiscuity to the female's desire for attention, for control, and to her inability to maintain healthy relationships, or, to the effects of bipolar disorder. (While the diagnostic criteria of promiscuous behavior during a manic episode is not gender-specific, it is extremely rare for this criteria to be applied to men.)

Nonmonogamous relationships are often viewed through a lens of assumed pathology with the perception that such relationships are inherently disturbed, as evidenced by the presence of sexuality with individuals outside the relationship. In 1997, two self-proclaimed "sluts," Dossie Easton and Catherine Liszt, turned the term upside down when they published a book that has since been vocally embraced by the nonmonogamous. *The Ethical Slut* served as a manifesto for those who had come to the realization that monogamy was simply not for them. The book explores the ins and outs (no pun intended) of nonmonogamous relationships, beyond just the "zipless fuck," Jong's anonymous sexual fantasy of the 1970s. While the book discusses the joys of group sex, orgies, public sex, cruising for partners, and the importance of health consciousness in such situations, it also goes well beyond these basic sexually driven topics. The book explores how to raise children when living this lifestyle, how to establish and protect healthy personal boundaries in any relationship, as well as how to enjoy and be skillful at sex. A central argument discusses the fear that love is based upon a starvation economy. According to this argument, we become jealous of our lovers' attention to others out of a fearful belief that there's only "so much to go around," and we lose out if our lover gives to others. In contrast, one might find pleasure in actually giving away that which others jealousy guard, the love and sexuality of their partner. Polyamorists call this "compersion," the pleasure they get from their partner's joy in love or sex with another.

A concern often raised about the swinging community is that it represents the expression of male fantasies about "no-strings attached" sex with others, and that women in this community are being forced to participate, or are being taken advantage of by their husbands. There is little research that focuses specifically upon the women involved in swinging, with most studies examining both partners. Historically, similar concerns have been raised about the negative effects of polygamy on women, notably among the polygamous marriages in Utah in the 1800s. More recent news stories about current polygamous families have focused upon the dominant power of the male in such relationships, and the ways in which some men have abused this power in marrying underage females and even engaging in sexual abuse of children.

Much of the research indicates that couples do typically enter swinging at the male's initial interest, but anecdotal reports and some limited research findings suggest that it is males who most often experience discomfort during swinging and suggest termination of swinging activities. The reason for this seems to relate to the importance of women in swinging, and the greater possibility that men will experience rejection within swinging. In other words, it is much more likely that men will have difficulty finding sexual partners, than will women. Swinging women have reported to researchers and in anecdotal accounts that they gain a boost to their ego through swinging, as they learn that they are attractive and desirable to others. But, studies examining ex-swingers do suggest that for couples that have dropped-out of swinging, the "wife's inability to take it" was frequently a significant factor in terminating their swinging, though jealousy, guilt, and marriage problems were far greater factors. Overall, women in swinging seem to report that they are generally happy with swinging, are happier with their relationships since they started swinging, and feel generally happier with their lives.

No research has indicated that swingers or especially swinging women were sexually abused as children or were/are victims currently. Many have suggested that such a history might make people prone to abnormal sexual behavior such as swinging, but this may reflect more of the bias against nonmonogamous relationships and uncommon sexual behaviors, rather than real evidence that individuals in swinging and nonmonogamous relationships have disturbed or traumatic sexual histories. Past research suggests that women in swinging were more likely to have been raised in laissez-faire families with little individual attention to the children's needs, but findings did not indicate any history of abuse.

Highly sexed women may sometimes find a level of acceptance and freedom in the culture around nonmonogamy, that they do not find in the rest of society. Psychologist Albert Ellis suggested that many women called nymphomaniacs were merely women with sexual drives comparable to men, and society attended to their sexuality only because of their gender. Gay Talese, author of *Thy Neighbor's Wife*, describing the sexual activities at the Sandstone commune, suggested that it was one of the first environments where highly sexed women could drop the need for feminine ploys and games, and merely pursue their sexual interests in a forthright and aggressive manner.[17]

The level of "normal" sexual interest in women continues to be a little understood phenomenon. In 2001, researchers Sandra Leiblum and Sharon Nathan published an article describing a rare, unknown disorder, wherein women reported persistent, unremitting sexual arousal. The five case studies the authors reviewed included the stories of women whose constant state of physiological sexual arousal led to tremendous difficulty concentrating and fulfilling daily activities. (This recalls to mind one of my wife's favorite jokes, regarding the woman who reports to a friend that she has strange condition that causes an orgasm each time she sneezes. Asked what she's taking for the problem, the woman replies, "Pepper.") However, while constant female sexual arousal might seem like a teenage boy's dream, these women reported that they were instead living a nightmare. Women profiled by Leiblum and Nathan identified symptoms of constant vaginal lubrication, clitoral and vaginal sensitivity, and physical arousal, only slightly and temporarily resolved by masturbation. These sensations and physical responsiveness were persistent, despite the women reporting no feelings of sexual desire that accompanied the physiological sensations. Although some research has continued with victims, there is little to no current explanation for the symptoms of what is now called "persistent sexual arousal syndrome."

In contrast, in 2008, Australian researcher Marita McCabe found that for 60 percent of the four hundred women she interviewed, a low level of sexual interest was the norm. Most women in her sample only experienced sexual interest when they were actually having sex. In other words, the chicken "came" before the egg did.

Whether or not females really hit a "biological peak" of sexuality around age thirty is unknown. There's little biological or physical evidence to support this theory. In the early 1900s, British sex researcher Havelock Ellis suggested that the "peaks" of female sexuality occurred between the years of twenty and thirty, and between the ages of forty and fifty, and mirrored the peaks of the onset of psychological disturbance, or "insanity."

Currently, it seems likely that this perceived "peak," when present or described, emerges from an older woman's increased sexual knowledge and confidence, and the increased ability to pursue one's own pleasure, within sexual activity, for the female. However, interestingly enough, infidelity appears to increase significantly for women, during the thirties and forties. Though these rates are changing somewhat, with increasing numbers of wives in their twenties admitting to infidelity, almost one-in-five women in their thirties has had extramarital sex, in contrast to less than one-in-ten in wives in their twenties.

Evolutionary theorists suggest that the alleged later sexual peak in females might reflect women having an urge to develop a "backup" plan of another potential mate, in the event that their current mate "dumps" them, as they've reached the end of their reproductive period. In the 1960s, sociologist Bernard Farber proposed that Westerners were moving towards a state of "permanent availability," whereby adults remained focused upon their own self-development and stability needs, maintaining a constant scanning of their social environment, for potential future mates and spouses. Another theory suggests that women in their late thirties are at the end of their fertile period, and aggressively pursuing the "genetically successful" male, to increase the likelihood of acquiring the males' genes to pass on to their children. It's interesting that research has shown that sexual satisfaction and fulfillment tops the list, when women are asked to identify the benefits they think they would get from an affair.

Motivations for female infidelity include factors related to sexual need, spontaneity, a woman's emotional well-being, and feelings of self-esteem. Dalma Heyn, author of *The Erotic Silence of the American Wife*, suggests that male infidelity is typically chalked up to biological urgencies, driven by impulse. Female infidelities are usually perceived as more calculated, more emotionally driven, and more indicative of problems within the woman or within the marriage. "I've always heard that's impossible—that a woman only has the capacity to love one man, and if she thinks she loves two, she probably doesn't love either," states a woman interviewed by Heyn.[18] Heyn's work suggests that the sexual reasons and the excitement of physical intimacies in female sexual infidelity, have been suppressed and kept secret, and that monogamy is treated as though it is a core female quality.

Estimates of female infidelity range, and it is generally accepted that infidelity, particularly by women, is underreported due to the social pressures upon women. Studies suggest that between 20 and 25 percent of women will have at least one outside sexual relationship during their marriage. Another quarter of women will have an intimate relationship, or fall in love with another person, though not pursue the relationship or allow it to become physical.

Recent studies suggest that the frequency of extra partner sex by women may be on the rise among younger women, to the point that the gender difference may actually disappear. A story called "Being unfaithful keeps me happy" was published in the British newspaper *The Telegraph*, and discussed the rising rates of female infidelity in Britain.[19] More and more, sexual infidelity is occurring among British wives, particularly among women who are successful and independent, and seeking sexual encounters with men other than their husband, simply because it feels good. One married, forty-three-year-old woman with two children and a very successful career said that "I am one of those women who want it all. My life is very hectic and I thrive on adrenaline. I really enjoy sex, but I don't want any complications. So I am only interested in men, preferably married, who want the same." Lynne, a forty-five-year-old business administrator told the reporter, "Now we are as successful as men at work and other areas of life, women like me think, 'Why the hell not?' My lover won't jeopardize my work or family life. I am doing something that makes me happy, which, in turn, makes home happier, too. Women have come a long way in the last twenty or thirty years, so why should taking a lover without commitment be a male preserve? I just think, 'Lucky me.'" Fifty-five-year-old Mary said "I've relearnt how to be a sexually confident woman, which is a good thing, and I also take much more care of my appearance." Not all of the women interviewed were merely seeking casual sex. Some sought emotional support they didn't get at home; others believed that it was impractical to expect one person to meet all their needs for the rest of their life.

Some women engage in infidelity as a revenge-seeking method, what is called "strategic infidelity." In contrast to males, who rarely cite revenge as a motivation for sexual infidelity, women often report that they have engaged in sexual infidelity as a means to punish their husband, sometimes for his own infidelity. Cuckold and hotwife stories are full of this, a plot device apparently based on true motivations. Straying husbands in these stories experience their wives' vengeance as the wives take their husbands' bosses, best friends, and enemies to bed. Numerous research studies have shown that when a person believes their spouse has been unfaithful, they are far more likely to themselves engage in subsequent infidelity.

Another factor in this increase in female infidelity in later life is that males are less likely to be intensely protective and restrictive over their wives, as they, and their marriages, reach this stage. This might occur for several reasons—first, the men might be preoccupied with looking for a younger female for themselves, and not really have the time to guard their wife. Also, by this time, the wife has probably already generated an heir or two for the husband, so protecting her might not be so important (in some historical cultures, there were documented periods where husbands of wives with many children sometimes "loaned" their wives out to other childless men, to assist the men in creating an heir). Domestic violence and spousal homicide are more common in couples with younger wives—the older the wife, the less frequent the arguing, and possessiveness of the husband, especially in cases where the wife's sexual fidelity is in question.

Studies have shown that the men whom women choose for illicit sex tend to be males who are more physiologically symmetrical, who are more likely to be evolutionarily successful, and often far more promiscuous. These men tend to have a history with the wives of other men—the higher the degree of measured facial symmetry in a male, the higher the number of married women he's taken to bed. These men are not the men that women should choose, if they're looking for a new, caretaking mate. But, if the goal is to increase the degree that a female's genes are passed on, having a child, particularly a son, by one of these males is a very effective strategy. A son who takes after his symmetrical, successful, and promiscuous father is apt to have far greater opportunities to pass on the genes inherited from his mother. This theory is sometimes called the "sexy son hypothesis."

Men with higher facial symmetry are often perceived by other men as being somewhat arrogant and forceful, and as sexier by women, particularly when women are ovulating. When women are not fertile, they often prefer men with softer faces, characteristics that might suggest a more sensitive personality. But, when ovulating, women are more drawn to men with stronger jaws and greater symmetrical features, evidence of higher testosterone and greater genetic potential.

Online, one man described how he had long tried to involve his wife in sex with other men, entreaties which she resisted. But, when his wife encountered a man she found extremely attractive, her husband's permissiveness took root. What the husband found surprising was that the man was not, to him, all that appealing. He described the man as having an "arrogant manner and commanding presence" which his wife found extremely seductive.[20] A wife similarly described a sexual encounter with an "arrogant and pushy" man, where the sex was extremely good, but after only one "romp" the wife sent the man away, something she described as a "first" for her.[21]

In 1974, sexuality researchers found that 18 percent of women reported enjoying fantasies of being with more than one man at the same time. Other studies have found similar rates, with figures that range between 10 and 41 percent of women endorsing erotic fantasies of having sex with two or more men at the same time, or, alternatively, one after the other. As evolutionary researchers Aaron Goetz and Todd Shackleford suggest, if "sexual fantasy provides a window through which to view evolved human psychology, then human female psychology may include design features dedicated to the pursuit of polyandrous sex, with the consequence of promoting sperm competition."[22]

Females, as compared to males, are far more capable of promiscuity. Kinsey, Fisher, and other notable anthropologists and sexual researchers have argued strongly that without the social risks, punishments, and prohibitions towards female promiscuity, women could and would far outstrip men in their level of promiscuity and multipartner sex. After ejaculation, males experience a refractory period, whereby they typically cannot perform sexually. Females experience no such break, are multiorgasmic, and almost infinitely receptive. Masters and Johnson suggested that females were able to have as many as fifty orgasms in a single session. In contrast, the greatest number of ejaculations by a male in a single session was between six and eight, by a male in Kinsey's data. Kinsey cited a male who was able to achieve twenty-one orgasms, in a twenty-four hour period. (Though I've got to say, this figure comes out of that creepy pedophilic data that Kinsey accepted, and which has always really, really disturbed me.) One of Mae West's young male lovers was reportedly able to reach twenty-six in a day's period. Experts do note that male ejaculation is not always synonymous with orgasm, and that some males can orgasm without ejaculation. Nonetheless, female orgasmic capacity so far outstrips that of males that we're really just arguing about a motor scooter chasing a Ferrari.

However, despite the female biological capacity for promiscuity, females are, according to most research, generally less interested than males in sex without relationship. Patricia Campbell, of Durham University, conducted a survey of 1,743 men and women, following "one-night stands," or dates that resulted in sex, without the development of a relationship. Men, as you might imagine, overwhelmingly reported feeling content and satisfied with the experience. In contrast with the 80 percent of males who were pleased with the experience, 54 percent of females viewed the experience as something positive and beneficial. The study's author described this as evidence that women are not as well-suited as men for uncommitted sex. But, I think the fact that over half of females actually enjoy a one-night stand is surprising, given the degree to which our society enforces the universal value that all women feel "cheap" and "used" after a one-night stand.

As women gain more sexual experience and confidence, more and more of them report having had sex with more than one man within thirty minutes of another. One study suggests that one in two hundred sexually experienced women have had this experience. One of twelve (about 8 percent) female college students have had a threesome with two men, and about 6 percent have had sex with more than two men at the same time.

Historically, wives have only been allowed sexual freedom in cultures where they controlled wealth or had political or economic independence. Most of the historical wives explored in this work were in upper-echelon economic categories, or were in the arts and literature, where female contributions to the arts have a longer history of acceptance. Research by Quaife into the legal records of seventeenth-century England does reveal that this practice has not been limited to the upper social strata. However, the fact that the majority of historical evidence for the practice is with regards to women in upper economic ranges suggests the possibility that, historically, it was these women who were freer to live this lifestyle openly. In today's greater sexual egalitarianism, the social prohibitions limiting this lifestyle to the rich and powerful may be eroding. The immense capacity of female sexual capacity is being quietly, but vigorously celebrated by some couples, who are not content to restrict the wife's sexuality within their marriage.

MICHELLE AND CHRIS

We're good people, nice people, not some freaks. We're in a loving committed relationship with one another and we happen to have lots of great sex with other people.

Michelle and her husband have lived a variety of nonmonogamous lifestyles for more than ten years. When Michelle first e-mailed me, she said they were looking forward to the opportunity to talk about their experiences. We had scheduled for me to interview them in my hotel suite, but working late threw them off schedule, and they asked if I could come to them, offering to meet in a coffee shop. I agreed, but was concerned that such a public setting might not readily support a useful interview. I shouldn't have worried.

Michelle and Chris were a biracial couple, he white and thirty-seven years old, and she black and twenty-nine years old. Chris was an intimidating looking man, with a muscular build, shaved head, prodigious beard, and large tattoos that blanketed his forearms. Once he warmed up, Chris displayed a generous nature, warm heart, and quick wit, and a bottomless wellspring of love for his wife.

Michelle is best described as vivacious. Sparks glinted from her flashing dark eyes and shining smile. She wore a clinging black dress that she frequently adjusted over her smooth legs and large, well-rounded bosom that heaved quite distractingly when she laughed, which was often. A surprising and compelling level of bedrock self-confidence was present in her every word and gesture. While she seemed to know how attractive she was, this awareness didn't seem to affect her much. Unlike some attractive women, I didn't notice her ever looking around, to see if she was getting the attention she was used to. She just went on, very comfortable with herself, and with receiving attention from those around her. She and her husband stayed close to each other, throughout the interview, and there was tremendous humor and respect for each other, in each word and story. Like many of the couples I met in this research, the depth and skill of their communication with each other was extremely developed, and they agreed that having been able to communicate and negotiate about their sexual issues had made any other problems pale by comparison.

Michelle and Chris met in Indiana, when he was twenty-three years old and she was fifteen. They both worked in retail stores, and Michelle apparently took a liking to Chris quite early on. Enough of a liking it seems, that she lied and told him she was eighteen. They became friends, and slowly worked up to dating over several months. It was only from her mother that Chris finally learned of her true age. Feeling that the age difference was too great, Chris broke up with Michelle, but maintained a platonic friendship for the next two years. They married shortly after Michelle turned eighteen. While they were "just friends," Michelle's mother passed away, and she recalled that she felt "trapped," living in the guardianship of her older siblings. On the day she turned eighteen, Chris came to the house, and Michelle left with him. They were married a few days later. A few months after they were married, Michelle told Chris that she was bisexual and had strong attractions for other women.

Michelle's first sexual relationships were with older women, and she had believed herself to be a lesbian for some time. Chris accepted this news calmly, with no defensiveness, merely asking what this meant for them. He didn't assume monogamy, and asked if it meant that she would have relationships with other women, and what his role would be in those relationships. Over time, they worked out boundaries, and eventually had a threesome with Michelle's best friend, who had never had sex with her, but was willing to explore the idea. Their relationship with this woman deepened over time, and the three lived together for some months, before parting ways. Following this, the couple decided to explore swinging, though they had to lie about Michelle's age, as most clubs don't allow individuals under twenty-one. However, Chris noted that with Michelle's confidence and sexiness, nobody ever questioned her age. At first, their relationships only involved other women, and Michelle shared how she was surprised by her first feelings of jealousy when watching her husband with another woman, but that these feelings quickly turned into pleasure. Likewise, Chris shared that the first time he saw Michelle with another man, he was hit in the gut by strong feelings, and was surprised to experience what she had felt while watching him with their female partners. But, as with Michelle, he said those feelings quickly turned into arousal.

Chris described his wife's personal and professional success with enormous pride, given that she had not completed high school or attended college, and felt that her business success was due to street smarts. He so enthusiastically described her success in spite of obstacles that Michelle blushed, which, given this woman's confidence and assuredness, seemed like a rare event.

As we sat in the coffee shop, we discussed their relationship, the couple describing how their marriage differed from relationships they had in the past, and those of people they knew. Chris commented "I had a girlfriend once, who found out my dad took me to a strip club, and she freaked out, over something so trivial. Why would I want to be with someone like that, where you have to lie?"

Michelle added, "We don't lie to each other. We don't have to lie about those things. We mostly do them together. There are some things, we do separately, Chris rides his motorcycle by himself, hangs out with the boys by himself. I hang out with the girls by myself. But most of the time, we do stuff together. I think that keeps us close-knit."

The open communication between the couple was clear, and extended beyond discussion of sexual issues. "I like the communication, together. If I spent twenty bucks, and I can tell her, I know she won't freak out. She can go shopping, and not have to hide stuff. I know men, and marriages, that are like that. If it's a money issue, we communicate a lot about finances, because they're really important," Chris said.

Michelle had only had "run of the mill boyfriends," before Chris, along with some older women that she had dated, when she briefly wondered if she was a lesbian. Chris was married once before, a short-lived marriage that happened "on a whim. We barely knew each other. Then she ended up cheating on me." Chris has seen lots of relationships around him, in his family and friends, crumble in response to infidelity. Chris's father has been married four times, and all of his previous marriages ended due to his father's infidelity. A few years ago, Chris and Michelle found out that Chris's father and his current wife are swingers as well. Chris said that he worries about the effects of infidelity, but feels that cheating is not an issue for him. The few times he's had sex without Michelle, he just called his wife, and told her about it. "She gets turned on by it. How is that cheating?"

Michelle agreed, "It's not cheating. Most of the time, we're together. Even when we're apart, it's not cheating, because I'm there with him."

Michelle leaned forward, her face alive, a brilliant white smile shining forth as she pumped her arm forward, saying, "Because I'll be on the phone, saying, 'Do it Baby, do it!'"

Chris smiled at his wife as she sat back in her seat, giggling. "Some of our ex-girlfriends have gone on to have relationships with men, and they got cheated on. Don't those men understand what they already have? Our girlfriend. . . ."

In that intensely synchronized communication style, so evident in this couple, Michelle interrupted, finishing Chris's thought. "She just found out yesterday."

Chris continued, "She found out yesterday, that her boyfriend, the father of her child, had been cheating on her the whole time she was pregnant." He laughed, in a tone that carried a tone of bitter surprise. "This was an ex-girlfriend of ours, she'd been with us, physically with us, for long periods of time. So, if this guy wanted something, on the side, she would have put it to him, super freaky. He could have had everything, his cake . . ."

Again, Michelle finished his thought, a smile on her face, "And eaten it too."

Chris finished his thought. "So, why cheat? He chose to be deceitful, when she would have given it to him, to put a smile on his face and give him a new experience. She did it with us, so why would he cheat? She would have sat back and coached him through the whole thing. I don't get it. It's mind-boggling."

"I used to have relationships without Chris, with other women, and sometimes men, but I don't too much anymore. At the beginning I did, but not so much anymore. Our enjoyment is together; it's not as good when he's not there. Although, Chris would like me to—he's turned on by me having sex with other people and coming home and telling him about it. Going out to meet a single man, it's an appealing thought to me, but not something I've done in a while. He would like for me to, he gets a kick out of it, but I don't," Michelle reached out and took her husband's hand.

Chris agreed, saying, "For me, the enjoyment is mostly about seeing the smile on her face, that's what is really important to me. I love the idea of her going out and hooking up with other guys, but I know it's not her thing, that gets her going. Why make somebody do something they don't want to do? That's what it comes down to."

Although Michelle said that Chris has permission to hook up with other women, and that she actually finds this exciting, Chris said that it happens rarely, as it is just "too much work, plus, after eleven years with Michelle, I could care less if another girl is interested or not."

Knowing that African Americans are not very visible in the swinging lifestyle, a group dominated by middle-class whites, I asked Michelle what her experience had been, given her ethnicity.

"Blacks are out there, in swinging, they're just not as public about it. What we've run into, they're not as public. They were usually raised in a religious atmosphere, have religious family members. They keep it very low-key and private. Most of our girlfriends are black women; we rarely have relations with a Caucasian female. There are lots of swinging black females, males, and couples, especially in the Midwest. Maybe not out here. Not many black people out here. They're there, but just not as out. I honestly think it's because of the religion. They were raised in a religious atmosphere and don't want to put their freaky thoughts out there. We are both spiritual people too but neither one of us practice a religion right now. I pray often and ask for forgiveness of my sins but that's about it. I don't agree with the whole 'God says you shouldn't' thing."

"It's a small town, and you feel like you're going to run into somebody at Wal-Mart, that's a freaky feeling. In Indiana, once, I ran into my elementary school principal there, in a swing club. I thought it was comical, he liked to run around in no pants, no underwear, just liked to be naked. I thought that was a bit too much for me, I had to go the other way," laughed Michelle.

Her husband laughed as well, "You could have fulfilled some of his fantasies!"

Michelle nodded, giggling and shaking in mirth, "But that would have messed me up just way too much, I mean, my grade-school principal?"

As close and intensely as this couple communicated, it was apparent that they know each other, about as well as two people can. They are rarely apart, and work together, in the same company, though Michelle acknowledged that even she was a little surprised how well it had worked out for them.

"Not all of our relationships are with women. We have been with couples, and the occasional single male. Most, like 89 percent have been with single women, the rest with couples and single men. Single males are very rare for us, because it's hard to find a single male, comfortable enough to be with a couple, and not be disrespectful with either of us. With a single female, she's usually more understanding, you can talk to her. She understands where we're both coming from. Being with a couple, I love it, being with couples. But it's hard to find couples, where you have chemistry, with both of them, and both of us. So, you have to make that chemistry between four people, as opposed to us and one other person, it's just a bit easier. I don't know any strangers, it's not that hard for me to meet people, but, Chris is a bit leery."

"With a guy, it needs to be right. If the guy is being arrogant and belligerent, I'm asking do I want this guy to be sexual with my wife when he's coming off condescending and arrogant? Why would I reward someone like that, when they've been disrespectful?" asked Chris. "Then there are the people that just want to have sex, but you're only attracted to one of them, and the other person does it, out of mercy. Has sex with someone they're not attracted to, so their partner can have sex with someone, like a 'come-along.' Where you're saying, wow, your wife is smoking, but your husband hasn't really taken care of himself, I'm not sure this is going to work out. Obviously you don't want to say that."

"Now, when we have a girlfriend and stuff, we try to help them realize they don't have to drink, to do it, that it's much better when you're sober, because you can feel it emotionally, as well as physically. It's a beautiful thing to us. It's perfectly normal to us, we're trying to figure out everybody else, and why on earth they cheat," said Chris.

"I think there would be less wars and less everything, if everybody was open and able to have a good time," added Michelle. "But, we're not up on the Internet every night trying to meet someone. It's not like that. We have a good relationship with each other, and if we meet someone that wants to come along, and we get along with them, it works out. We do just fine by ourselves. We rehash the old times sometimes, but do just fine by ourselves. We've rarely gone more than a month without being with somebody."

"It's almost becoming a part of who we, Chris and Michelle, are," said Chris.

"Our friends know us like that. We have friends that are in monogamous relationships, couldn't possibly see themselves in the lifestyle. They understand what we do, but would never do it. I understand, it's not meant for everybody," said Michelle. "We don't surround ourselves with people that would judge us, shake their finger at us, tell us we're going straight to hell. Some family members. My aunt is married to a pastor. She found out, I was out somewhere with our first girlfriend, my best friend, and it came out. Her response to it was that you guys are going to burn in hell. Brimstone and fire. It was negative for a while, she told other family. It got ugly for a minute. But then she began to understand that he's not going out and doing it with other people, without my knowledge. Once she understood better, and I could communicate with her, it was okay."

Chris smirked a bit, his bald head shining, long beard wiggling, "I'm not that approachable, people don't come at me like that."

"We do have friends and family that object to this, they don't understand why we do this, and how? They say it's just like cheating and don't understand how I can know he's not going to fall in love with someone else," said Michelle. "I explain to people that I know he's never going to find another me, nobody else can give him what I give him, so I don't worry about it. And we have sex with other people, I make love to him, that's a big difference to me. Having sex with somebody is just run of the mill, him, I'm with for the rest of my life."

"You put emotion into it, and have fun with it, but that person you just had sex with, you're not going to talk to them about balancing the checkbook or paying the bills, the important things. Sex is an expression of how we enjoy ourselves, with each other and other people. Other people go bowling, this is what we do, and I have to drink Gatorade to recover from it sometimes," laughed Chris.

"We always have a friend, it's weird to say, but we've made lots of friends in this lifestyle," added Michelle.

"We're not out having random sex with people we just met, in bathrooms and such. That's okay," Michelle paused for a moment, a wicked little smile on her face. "Sometimes, that's more than okay, but we're not doing it, at least, not anymore.

"I've always wanted to tell my story, share, tell the true experience of my relationship, not just the sex, not just that I'm bisexual and we're swingers. I want to tell my story. We're good people, nice people, not some freaks. We're in a loving committed relationship with one another and we happen to have lots of great sex with other people."

Chris nodded vigorously, agreeing with his wife, and then looked intensely at me. Staring into his dark eyes, I had an odd juxtaposition, seeing this man at once as the fearsome looking biker he presented himself as, and at the very same moment, as a very sensitive and loving husband who cared deeply for his wife, and for the feelings of others. "The fact of getting the story out, as we did this, not once have you been judgmental, sat back and said you could never do that. We get that with other people, which is why we don't talk about it usually, but, we're not embarrassed about it."

"Not at all. We're open about it. There are a lot of worse things. Even in this town, especially in this town, there are worse things than Chris and Michelle," Michelle said.

Chris's disclosure about his father's infidelity, and participation in swinging raises an intriguing issue. Chris was apparently aware of his father's infidelity, but only became aware of his father's involvement in swinging long after Chris himself was in the swinging lifestyle. Some anecdotal research with swingers has suggested that there are some family connections, with some individuals being introduced to swinging via their parents' activities. But a more intriguing question is whether nonmonogamous behaviors may be heritable, either through genetics, child-rearing environment, or both. Indeed, studies with twins have shown that infidelity has a high heritability rate of around 40 percent. This means that in twins, if one twin has a history of infidelity, it is a 40 percent chance that the other twin has also engaged in extramarital sex. The heritability rates of bipolar disorder and schizophrenia, two of the most heritable, clearly genetically linked mental disorders, have similar heritability rates around 59 percent and 46 percent, respectively.

Sexologist Dr. Marty Klein argues that growing anecdotal and research evidence suggests that "kinkiness" and nonmonogamy may be more akin to sexual orientation, with a heritable, biological origin and lifelong stability. Many couples involved in swinging, hotwifing, and cuckoldry shared with me that their parents were not monogamous either. Some individuals discovered this as children while others did not learn it till they were already adults and rejecting monogamy themselves.

I corresponded with a Texas physician, nicknamed Princess, who was involved in the hotwife lifestyle. She described finding pictures and videos of her parents having sex with other people, when she was teenager. When she found the videos, and watched her mother on the television, having sex with men other than her husband, Princess realized that the messages about waiting until marriage, and only having sex when you're in love, were a "load of crap." A few weeks later, Princess lost her virginity to a neighborhood boy. She described that she felt relatively disappointed by the sex with this boy, but then had sex with his older brother, and found that "experience really does make a difference." Princess's mother caught her with one of these boys, and the maternal relationship changed forever.

> I just stood there, my blouse still open with her screaming at me, but then she got quiet and just stared at me. I finally broke the silence and told her she had a lot of guts to scream at me for [having sex with] Matt and confronted her about their pictures and videos. The balance of power shifted big time but put us on equal footing. We sat down and had our first real adult sexual conversation and she explained that she and my stepfather were swingers and what swinging was all about. I asked her if they didn't get jealous of each other and she explained not only no, but how much it turned each one on to see or know of them [having sex with] someone else. I have been very sexually active since that day and never had to hide it from mom and my step dad again.[1]

Sociologist Lynn Atwater has suggested that the increasing availability of mothers and wives to be sexual beings, fulfilling their own sexual desires may also increase the degree to which these women are able to educate their daughters about sexuality. Atwater suggests that these women, like the mother of the teenaged Princess, may be better able to discuss with their daughters how to define sexuality for themselves, and how to find pleasure in sexuality, beyond the traditional maternal messages about sexuality, including safety, chastity, and monogamy. Dalma Heyn has pointed out that usually, the only sex education mothers offer their daughters concerns how to be safe and how to be nice; rarely do daughters hear about how to experience sexual pleasure, or assert one's sexual needs in a healthy way. Perhaps, as more women assert themselves sexually, these social discussions of female sexuality will prompt more mother-daughter conversations about these topics.

4

ALTERNATIVES TO MONOGAMY

Hard work is damn near as overrated as monogamy.

Huey Long[1]

When one considers the seeming universality of the expectation of monogamy in today's world, it is perhaps surprising that monogamy has not always been the expected state for man. Despite the vehemence with which many Christians defend monogamy, many in the Bible, including David and Solomon, were far from monogamous. Throughout the history of man, most societies practiced a range of relationships, with monogamy and polygyny (a marriage arrangement with one man and multiple wives) the most common, with only rare societies that mandated monogamy. Currently, less than 20 percent of world cultures require monogamy, the overwhelming majority allowing polygamous marriages. Less common were societies that practiced polyandry, where one woman has multiple husbands (which reportedly were found in less than 1 percent of worldwide societies). In as many as 40 percent of world societies, currently and throughout history, according to some anthropological studies, extramarital sexual activity is not prohibited, but is in fact encouraged by social rules and guidelines. Some cultures considered it polite for a man to share his wife with other men, and others supported extramarital sex with certain people or at certain times like holidays or during fertility rites. In 1867, traveler Thomas Lawson described an event in the Marquesas

Islands, where a single woman reportedly had sex with 103 different men over a single night, during a cultural ritual.

In an ancient Hindu Sanskrit tale, Mahabharata, a female character named Draupadi marries five brothers. Draupadi is a princess, and betrothal to her is to be earned in a contest of archery. The brothers, along with other suitors compete, and one of the brothers, Arjuna, succeeds in the contest, securing Draupadi to be his bride. When the brothers return home, they tell their mother to see what Arjuna won. In the timeless tradition of mothers around the world, their mother tried to avoid sibling conflict. Without looking, she told the brothers to share whatever had been won, and thus, following their mother's orders, all five brothers married Draupadi.

Not all early cultures took aggressive, murderous views of adultery. In some North American tribal cultures, a man cuckolded by his wife would challenge the other man to a singing contest. In other tribal cultures, the man simply took the other man's wife in place of his own, as an exchange of sorts. In some Inuit traditions, a husband might willingly share his wife with a male guest, though this occurred less than urban myth might lead us to believe. Certainly, this was not a case of men sharing their wives with every Tom, Dick (ahem), and Harry who appeared at the front door. Monogamy was not universally practiced or expected in Inuit tradition, and some relationships were explicitly open, at the request of both husband and wife. And yes, sometimes the husband would willingly share his willing wife with other men. However, according to anthropologists, the practice of wife trading served several very specific cultural roles. It occurred within formal boundaries, with defined relationships.

Inuit husbands who shared their wives with other men called the other man "Aipak," which meant "another me." Children of the two families referred to each other as "katuk," or half-sibling. Children referred to their parents' partners as "Aaparuk" or "Aanaruk," or little father or little mother. Sharing each other's wives served as a form of contract between two men, showing their commitment to each other. This role served to facilitate economic and social support between the two men; when one man was killed or challenged, his "wife-trading partner" was expected to step forward to defend, or avenge him. Because strangers were feared, and often killed outright, when men traveled the lands, the relationships and children created by trading wives back and forth served to extend familial bonds across tribes and distance. At least one significant historical battle between tribes was stopped, when participants acknowledged that their parents had traded wives, and thus, the potential combatants had a formal familial relationship and could not be enemies.

In some Inuit tribes, the practice of wife trading occurred with a formalized exchange between the two men. One might comment that the other's wife was pretty. If the other responded that he also thought the other man's wife was pretty, then an exchange of wives had been agreed to. However, if the husband simply agreed that yes, his wife was pretty, it was a polite way of telling the man that the trade was not going to happen. Among the Siberian Tschuktschi, before a male guest could enjoy the company of his host's wife, he had to swish his mouth with a cup of the woman's urine, to display his boldness and manliness, and as a form of commitment to the family. Thus did he show himself as a friend of the family. In the Ammassalik tribe of the Arctic, husbands offered their wives sexually to a guest by playing what they called the "putting out the lamp game." By putting out the oil lamp at night, the husband was implicitly allowing his wife to have intercourse with their guest. However, it must be noted that this wasn't free reign for the wife—if she was caught having sex with the guest at other times, without the husband's "putting out the lamp," she could be severely punished, and her lover even killed by her angry, jealous husband. This limitation was present in many of the Inuit and Arctic tribes' practices of wife sharing.

Jealousy and infidelity were not unknown in the Inuit culture, and often resulted in the same sorts of bloody violence present across other cultures. Jealousy is often present, even prevalent, in current incidents of spousal violence among the modern Inuit, especially among incidences of a husband actually murdering their wife, something that sadly occurs at high rates among current Inuit populations. Rules had to be followed, and sex outside the marriage that did not follow those rules could and did result in dramatic violence and death, of the wife or the lover. Sometimes, though, husbands could use the rules, and pretend they had been followed, to avoid a conflict. In some cases recounted by Lawrence Hennigh, husbands who found their wives had been with other men, outside the confines of established wife sharing, sometimes chose to act as though the acts had been sanctioned, calling the other man "Aipak," and offering consent after the fact.

So-called "civilized" men did sometimes take advantage of these customs. One story describes a physician who lived amongst a Sioux tribe, and took advantage of Chief Spotted Tail's offer of his wife. However, that physician, who reportedly had a very attractive wife of his own, was quite perturbed when the Chief asked him to "return the favor" so to speak. No word, of course, about how either the Chief's or the physician's wife may have felt about this arrangement.

Sexual jealousy over one's wife may have been relatively uncommon in preindustrial cultures. Wives, in many cases, were viewed more as property, and infidelity yielded jealousy and anger over the loss of control and sole possession of a valuable commodity, rather than what we know today as sexual jealousy, and the specific emotion around guarding and protection of sexual activity. As with the Inuit, the practice of "sharing" one's wife or wives with honored guests was present in many other cultures, in North and South America, Micronesia, Polynesia, Asia, India, Africa, and among indigenous Australians. In the Sandwich Islands, visitors were offered full hospitality by their hosts, which included the opportunity to bed their hosts' wives or even daughters.

Customs around this sharing and hospitality varied dramatically, between tribes and cultures, even within close geographical proximity and cultural origins. In some areas of the Middle East, where a guest might be free to caress and kiss the wife of their host, the guest would be instantly slain if he took the opportunity further. In other areas of the same region, there were no such constraints placed upon the guest.

In most, if not all, of these cases of wife sharing as a form of hospitality, the decision and control lay with the husband. Indigenous Australian men might offer their wife to a guest, but would aggressively punish unsanctioned adultery, or advances by other men, when they occurred outside his control. In some of these Australian tribes, a wife could approach her husband for permission to sleep with another man, permission that was often granted. Among the same tribes, it was often the custom for older brothers to share their wives with younger brothers, understanding that later, when the younger brothers had married, the older brothers would have the favor returned. Among Native Americans in early California, the choices of wives who slept with men of their husband's family were accepted, but condemned if the other man was unrelated to the husband.

Polygyny, the practice of males having multiple female mates or wives, has been common throughout the world's history, and is a reproductive strategy that has been reserved for the most successful, powerful males in societies. The reverse, polyandry, where females have multiple male mates, has been exceptionally rare. The few known instances have typically involved females married to male siblings. Thus, the brothers could share a female, knowing that the children carry their genes, whether they come from one brother or another. This was the case in some areas of the East, notably Tibet, Nepal, and Ceylon. Fraternal polyandry, where brothers marry a single woman, was practiced in some areas of India as well. Fraternal polyandry also served an economic function, by conserving family wealth and the inheritances of brothers, and ensuring the care and support of children within the family. In Tibet, as many as four to six men, usually brothers, would sometimes marry a single woman. The family lived in harmony, with established rules and protocols that governed the "sharing" of the wife. It is noteworthy that polyandry has been more common in societies where females controlled significant wealth, comparable to the prevalence of polygyny in societies where a few men controlled a significant portion of the economic resources.

A form of fraternal polyandry is somewhat more common, defining a practice in which females are shared by males who are genetically related to each other, such as brothers. Among gorillas, a species where single males usually jealously rule over a harem of females, a version of fraternal polyandry is sometimes practiced, as brothers and sons sometimes share a group of female gorillas. Fraternal polyandry was practiced by ancient Jews, as Israelite society practiced "levirate marriage," where the brother-in-law of a widow was sometimes required to marry the wife of his deceased brother. In some traditions, if the widowed woman had no living male children, the brother-in-law was expected to have sex with her. If a child was conceived, the child was considered to be the child of her deceased husband. A description of this practice is given in the Bible, in Deuteronomy.

Around 2300 BC, Urukagina of Lagash, King of Sumeria, decreed that all women who married multiple men were to die by stoning. Polyandry had been a common practice in the land before Urukagina's pronouncement. Urukagina is known as history's first government reformer, and the originator of the first formal legal code in human history. It seems somehow noteworthy that one of the first acts of government reform was to order the stoning deaths of women who married more than one man.

Many societies have included times of acceptable female promiscuity, often around fertility festivals, where women copulated with multiple males. Anthropologically, this is likely to have been a social strategy that promoted the continuation of the tribe, ensuring that males protected the woman's children, even after the woman's primary mate may have died in warfare or hunting. In some societies this was formalized, as a part of the culture, with terms, patterns of relationships, and ethics that defined and governed the nonmonogamous behaviors. "Partible paternity" refers to the practice of more than one male sharing degrees of fatherhood of a woman's child.

In the Bari tribe of Venezuela, who live in an extremely resource-poor environment, most pregnant women deliberately have sex with other tribal males. With their husbands' full knowledge and consent, the pregnant women seek out additional men in the tribe for sexual encounters. These encounters seem to primarily occur only after the woman is pregnant, but, after delivering her child, the midwife goes to tell each of the woman's lovers that they now have a child. These secondary mates have formal, socially defined protective roles to play with regards to the woman's child, increasing the assurance of the protection of that child, and the tribe's continuation. Granted, the husbands in the Bari are not monogamous either, as they are having sex with the other pregnant wives in the tribe. One can imagine that this would generate an intense community of intertwined parental and care-giving obligations, which would support the overall future of the tribe, and increase the chances that any individual male's children would survive. Indeed, research by anthropologists has shown that Bari children with more than one "father" have a significantly greater chance of surviving to adulthood. In a newspaper article by Karen Freeman, anthropologist Stephen Becker reported that he also asked if Bari women deliberately looked for lovers after they became pregnant so their children would have better food to eat. "After the laughter died down," he said, "one of them put her arm around my shoulder and said, 'Steve, I don't know how it is with your people, but among us, it's the boys who chase the girls.'"[2]

In another South American tribe, the Ache of Paraguay, anthropologists Kim Hill and Hillard Kaplan reveal that Ache women have three different types of fatherhood, referring to the man the woman was married to, the men she had sex with before and during her pregnancy, and the man that she believes is actually the biological father of her child.

The woman depends upon each man to protect and provide for her and her children. In both the Ache and the Bari, there is little jealousy or conflict reported around the nonmonogamous behavior of the wives.

The Kuikuru, an extremely small Amazonian tribe, have an accepted pattern of extramarital sexual relationships, by both husbands and wives. The Kuikuru reportedly marry at a young age, and throughout their lives, take "ajois," or outside lovers. The Kuikuru use friends and social relationships to arrange their extramarital sexual relationships, and the ajois relationships play a valuable, socially important role in the tribe. According to Robert Carneiro, the anthropologist who studied the Kuikuru, most of the adult tribe members have numerous lovers outside their marriage, sometimes as many as ten. Divorce in the Kuikuru is very easy and nonconfrontational—often, one spouse simply takes their belongings and moves into a different hut or house, or even into a different portion of their house, to establish a formal break in the marriage.

In ancient Rome and Sparta, when a man had enough children, he would sometimes offer his wife to other men, who desired children. Though there were strict rules against female adultery in Rome, wives sometimes renounced their family name and registered as prostitutes, sometimes with their husband's consent, as a way to circumvent the laws against female infidelity. Women who were registered as prostitutes could not be punished for their sexual acts, even if they were married.

In ancient Germany, if a man was impotent, or otherwise unable to impregnate his wife, he would sometimes invite another man into her bed. Martin Luther wrote, in recognition of this tradition:

> Then suppose I should further counsel her, with the consent of the man (who is not really her husband, but merely a dweller under the same roof with her), to give herself to another, say her husband's brother, but to keep this marriage secret and to ascribe the children to the so-called putative father. The question is: Is such a woman in a saved state? I answer, Certainly. Because in this case the error and ignorance of the man's impotence are a hindrance to the marriage; the tyranny of the laws permits no divorce; the woman is free through the divine law, and cannot be compelled to remain, continent. Therefore the man ought to yield her this right, and let another man have her as wife whom he has only in outward appearance.[3]

In eighteenth-century Turkey, polygamy and the keeping of harems was common. Many men had multiple wives and concubines. Women wore full coverings and veils in public, and one might thus assume that this culture, male-dominated as it might seem, would take great lengths to prohibit female adultery. Surprisingly, the Lady Mary Wortley Montagu, a traveler and writer, pointed out that veils and full coverings actually served to assist the Turkish women in their frequent and common infidelities. She suggested an unfaithful wife could walk down the street with her lover, right past her husband, and, because of the veils, was anonymous and safe. Further, because these women were often independently rich, they had a freedom that Montagu described as unique and unprecedented in Europe.

Droit de Seigneur, also known as *jus primae noctis*, or "first night," is the supposed medieval custom whereby a feudal noble could claim the right to sleep with a serf's wife on the first night of their marriage. Despite the drama, and the cuckoldry-inspired tragic elements of such a custom, there is little evidence that such a custom was widely practiced in the Middle Ages.

The French writer and philosopher Voltaire argued that the right of the first night was a form of social tyranny that was never legally or formally sanctioned. However, given the fear of cuckoldry in the Middle Ages, one can certainly imagine the political usefulness that such a rumored custom might have for those who opposed the power of the nobility.

Practices similar to the first night occurred in other cultures, often in rituals where the wife was first offered to the priest or religious leader. In Troy, legend holds that women would bathe in a sacred river before their wedding night, symbolically rendering their virginity to the god of the river. According to some legends, young men would sometimes masquerade as that same god, deflowering the young bride physically, as well as symbolically. In Greece, religious rites were sometimes abused, as priests masqueraded as gods who claimed the privilege of deflowering the wives. In Rome, ancient Roman chieftains took it as their right to deflower new brides, and even charged the groom a fee for doing so. Later, civil laws gave the Roman emperor legal access to sex with any Roman citizen's wife, a legal right that some emperors took advantage of, for political purposes. The scholar Augustine noted that some Roman brides would sit on the throne of Priapus, which featured a large phallus, and ostensibly removed the woman's modesty at the least, and perhaps her virginity. Some cultures held that the blood from the breaking of a woman's hymen was dangerous to a male, and so other women or sometimes religious leaders were delegated to perform this duty, prior to the couple's first night together. Marco Polo described that in Tibet, men were reluctant to marry women who could not prove a history of sexual promiscuity, under the assumption that such women were thus more attractive and skilled in bed. Polo shared that the region was perfect for a young man to travel in, as he would find many young women who sought to bed him, in order to increase their status. Even in ancient Christian weddings, some rites allowed the priest to kiss not only the bride, but all the women in the wedding party, before the husband could legally kiss his wife (though as previously described, once betrothed, premarital sex was, in fact, quite common). Alternatively, the bride was sometimes expected to kiss all the men of the husband's family. Some historians suggest that the line "You may now kiss the bride" is a vestige of this tradition.

In some southern Slav cultures, wives would offer themselves sexually to their new husband's male relatives, or even sometimes to all males at the wedding. Some semblance of this practice still continues, in symbolic fashion. Among many traditional and American immigrant cultures, the "money dance" is an event held at the wedding reception, where men offer money to the groom or his best man in order to dance with the bride. This custom appears to have originated in Poland in the 1900s, and is used as a way for guests to offer the new couple money with which to start their lives together. While the tradition has no direct connection to the history of wife sharing in other cultures, it does seem a symbolically similar ritual.

In many stories and celebrations of the cuckold fetish, this ritual is acted out in erotic form, wherein the groom loses his wife on their wedding night, to sexual encounters with other, more dominant men. These husbands also often celebrate the image of their wives still wearing their wedding rings as they touch another man sexually, with that ringed hand. One husband described online that though he and his fiancée had intended to have her take her vows, while her vagina was filled with the semen of other men, they were unable to accomplish this due to the complexities of wedding logistics. Instead, she "visited" with another man during the reception, and then danced with her husband, telling him while they danced, that another man's semen was running down her legs.

> In a way, the fantasy I like even more is my wife sleeping with another man the night before our wedding. The idea of standing next to her and taking our vows while knowing his [semen] is inside her is a huge turn on for some reason.
>
> Over the years I've learned that three men attending our small wedding had gone to bed with my wife at one point or another (including a guy who still sleeps with her from time to time). I like going through our wedding album, seeing their pictures, and knowing that, as they watched the ceremony, all they were probably thinking about were the times they had sex with my bride. Their [semen] was in her that day in spirit, if not in fact.[4]

The swinging culture is referred to by many engaged in it as "the lifestyle." Both a book and a movie have been written under this name, both depicting the people and practices of married men and women who pursue sexual interactions with others, with the explicit consent and approval of their spouses. There is some debate about the origins and history of this lifestyle, with some relating it to military marriages, others describing the possibly apocryphal "key parties" of the 1960s, where the men placed their keys into a bowl and the wives went home as sexual partners of the man whose keys they drew from the bowl. According to most of those writing about swinging, it surged in popularity in the 1970s, nosedived in the 1980s with the rise of HIV, and has resurfaced with increasing popularity in the past decade.

Swinging usually happens at clubs, or between couples who meet through advertisements in magazines and on the Internet. There are currently swing clubs in every state in the United States, as well as many international clubs throughout most geographic regions. Swing clubs and activities have become much more public in recent years, as the revenues and business associated with them has grown. Regular lifestyle conventions and conferences occur in hotels and resorts across the world. Such clubs and gatherings generate millions of dollars in revenues, as couples and individuals fork over hundreds and thousands of dollars to attend and participate. While there has been more research about swingers than any other nonmonogamous group, much of this research is dated, with little empirical research in the past two decades. Books and movies about the lifestyle have been written, by both those in and out of the swinging community, exploring the practices and characters of swingers. These pieces tend to be polemic, either arguing strongly for the benefits of swinging, or presenting the ugly and tawdry sides of the lifestyle. In both research and popular media, the presentation of swingers and the questions about them are strongly affected by the values and approaches of those leading the investigation.

In 1999, journalist Terry Gould published a book about his year in *The Lifestyle.* He explores the community of swingers, and interviews couples who pursue nonmonogamous sexual activities with others. His book, a national best-seller, documented discussions of the history of swinging, and the intense sexual politics that occur within and around swinging couples. Gould presents compelling examples of the power and respect that women within swinging have, in contrast to the academic and social belief that swinging is about the fulfillment of male desire, through subjugation of female autonomy.

Much of Gould's book focuses upon the women in swinging, and their reported enjoyment and empowerment through nonmonogamous sexual activity with their husbands. Over and over, he described women who were regarded as anomalous at the least, or disturbed at the worst, due to their strong sex drives, sex drives that they had little interest in restraining. Gould suggests that "sperm competition syndrome," an evolutionary concept explored in detail in chapter 10 of this work, explains the intensity with which husbands respond to their wives' sexual interactions with other men.[5]

Open marriage was most clearly defined as a concept by Anna and George O'Neill in their book of the same name, published in the 1970s. Although the term now denotes couples who "have an arrangement" to allow sexual relationships outside their marriage, this was only a limited component of the O'Neills' relationship concept. The O'Neills argued that the expectation that the two partners in a couple could completely meet each other's needs is a generally unhealthy and destructive expectation that "closes" and inhibits the growth of both individuals. The authors argued that many couples would be healthier if they were able to step outside of the personal, cultural, and gender-role expectations they bring to their marriage. This would allow, for instance, each partner to have outside friendships and growth experiences, with the idea that such growth would strengthen the marriage by increasing the personal growth of each partner in the marriage. That such outside relationships might become sexual was only a part of the O'Neills' premise, but it was this controversial idea that caught the greatest public attention. The O'Neills offered sexually open marriages as a way to address the growing prevalence of infidelity, and the devastating effects it had upon marriages. They argued that fidelity is best defined as the commitment partners have to one another, to each other's growth as well as to their own, rather than an allegiance to a sexual obligation.

Many of the things the O'Neills advocated actually came to pass, with social acceptance of more flexible gender roles in relationships as more married women entered the workplace. Today's relationships are more acknowledging of the individual's commitment to personal growth within their relationship. A backlash of sorts has now occurred, with a plethora of books available now that trumpet the warning signs of "emotional infidelity," and warn spouses about the dangers of their husbands or wives having friendships that "take away" from the marriage. Now that females have more freedom and latitude in society, it is impossible for a man to constantly assure his wife's sexual fidelity when she is away from him. As a result, the restrictions and limitations once put upon physical intimacy are now being expanded, and placed upon relationships of all kinds, to prevent spouses from developing friendships that are too risky, or too close. Author Dalma Heyn has suggested that we have deified truth telling, in requiring truth and honesty from our spouses as a measure of love. In fact, that truth telling may merely be a means by which spouses exert greater control over each other.

Little research and writing has been done about open marriages specifically. While the term was identified in some research, separate from swinging, and is still found in some demographic research about sexual practices, few empirical studies have addressed the characteristics of this group. In current writing, most include open marriage in another category of nonmonogamous relationships, polyamory.

Patricia Dorsky was living an experimental open marriage with her husband David in the 1970s when author Linda Wolfe interviewed her. At the age of twenty-four, Patricia was college-educated and a successful executive for a clothing company. According to Wolfe's interview with Patricia and David, her husband instigated the openness and nonmonogamy of their marriage, to assist Patricia during a period of depression, when she was "feeling unattractive and rotten and stupid. Nothing about other men or women happened until I was going through a period when I was very depressed. I'm a depressive type."[6] Her husband David, knowing Patricia was feeling this way, encouraged her to spend time with a man he had met, saying "You would really like Jan."[7] One night, at a party, Patricia found that she did indeed like Jan. The three stayed up late together, until David fell asleep on the couch, and Jan and Patricia "got into his bed and fooled around and then made it."[8] Patricia struggled with Jan though, in that as she wanted to continue the relationship, with David's encouragement. Jan was reluctant, concerned that David must not love Patricia, and he did not want to be a part of marital conflict or the relationship's demise. Eventually, Patricia was able to encourage Jan to seek, and acquire, David's permission. Jan then asked if Patricia was doing this because she didn't really love David, to which Patricia responded that she loved him very much and had no intention of leaving him. Patricia saw Jan often, though somewhat irregularly, sometimes as many as three times a week, and sometimes only once.

Jan was moody and depressive, like Patricia, but she felt that she could never marry a man like him. David accepted Patricia, despite her depression, and her tendency to lash out, acceptance that she never felt from Jan. Patricia explained that she initially worried that David was jealous of her relationship with Jan, and wasn't telling her or admitting it. Finally though, she decided "he really isn't jealous because he knows that our relationship is something that can't be touched by anyone else. He knows that I don't like people terribly much and that it's rare for me to meet someone that I want to be involved with."[9] Sex with Jan was special, because of the feeling of "newness," a feeling that had been lost with David.

When Wolfe interviewed David, she noted that David was emphatic that he was not homosexual. Nor was he trying to get rid of Patricia, by foisting her off on another man. David "thought another relationship would be good for her at this time and he figured that nothing that ever happened with other men would come between them."[10] David himself was not involved in any outside relationships, and said that it just wasn't really worth the work it would require.

Polyamory emerged as a defined concept in the 1990s, spurred by the Internet, growing from discussions of "responsible nonmonogamy," and including concepts of open marriages, communal living, and sexual freedom. The book *Stranger In A Strange Land*, by Robert A. Heinlein is one of the more popular books among the polyamory community, with its exploration of group marriage and nonpossessive relationships. Similarly, *The Harrad Experiment*, by Robert Rimmer, a Harvard Business School graduate, depicted a utopian sexual environment of open, group marriages on a university campus. Rimmer and his wife Erma maintained a stable sexual relationship for years, with another couple. It was this experience that led him to write *The Harrad Experiment*, and he was reportedly quite surprised to find that he and his wife and partners were not the only ones in America with such desires.

Robert A. Heinlein, whose science fiction books inspired much of the current polyamory movement, was, according to writer Isaac Asimov, a nudist who had an open marriage with his second wife, Leslyn. In 1942, Asimov was invited to Heinlein's home, and later recalled Heinlein proudly using a projector to display photographs of his nude wife to Asimov and their fellow writers. In *Stranger in a Strange Land*, Heinlein wrote:

> There's no need for you to covet my wife . . . love her! There's no limit to her love, we all have everything to gain—and nothing to lose but fear and guilt and hatred and jealousy.[11]

Polyamory means "many loves," and rejects the idea that a person can truly love only one person at a time. It is a broad concept, encompassing many different relationship types and approaches. It is conceived as a growth from the open marriages, group marriages, and sexual explorations of the past decades. The polyamory movement sets few limits upon relationships, other than expecting people to be responsible and honest with their relationships, both within and without monogamy. Polyamorous relationships and sexual encounters can include both partners in a couple, as in swinging or group marriages, but more often resemble open marriages, with one or both partners having external relationships. Specific language and terms have arisen around the unique aspects of polyamory, to describe the relationships, such as the term "vee" to describe a relationship between three people where one person (the point of the vee) has an intimate relationship with both other people (the legs of the vee), but the two other individuals in the relationship do not have an intimate relationship with each other. Some writers and proponents distinguish it from polyfidelity, wherein a group of more than two people establish a commitment to monogamy within the group, eschewing sexual relationships with those outside the group.

Polyamory is primarily defined through books and articles written by its proponents, especially through the electronic medium of the Internet. There has been relatively little research on the polyamorous, save as they may be included in research with swingers, or as researchers have examined polyamory in homosexual couples. Most of those writing about or researching polyamory are individuals who are themselves interested in or living polyamorous lifestyles. There is an ongoing debate within the polyamorous community as to whether or not relationships based solely upon sex should be included as forms of polyamory. Many strive to differentiate polyamory from swinging, highlighting its emphasis upon love, relationships, and honesty, rather than the sexual focus of swinging.

Many swingers report establishing long-lasting intimate friendships with their swing partners, and many who identify as polyamorous engage in sexual adventures and relationships with others. As in sexual orientation, there are a wide range of behaviors and relationships associated with the identity of those who call themselves polyamorous. Much of the research that has been conducted with polyamorists indicates that many have participated in sexual play parties or sex-only relationships, despite their stated orientation towards love-based relationships.

Interestingly, stigma is applied within the different groups who practice nonmonogamy, as much as it is applied against them. Andrew, whose story is told in the first interlude, shared with me that while he and his wife identify as polyamorous, they have to keep the details of their sexual practices secret, or face judgment from polyamorists who feel there is not enough love and relationship in their sexual encounters. Those who practice cuckoldry and hotwifing also experience rejection from swingers, who find their sexual practices to be bizarre and deviant:

> It never ceases to amaze me at how prejudiced participants in other forms of the "swinging lifestyle" are of cuckold couples. It is worse than

the vanilla population's treatment of "swingers", which that vanilla population paints with one brush. . . .

Why? Because most people think of "swinging" as a "couple who has sex with other couples." The idea that a husband would "allow" his wife to have other lovers, while not enjoying the same "freedom" would be even more shocking, I would think.[12]

What is a hotwife? Not surprisingly, *Webster's* doesn't define it. Wikipedia defines a hotwife as a subculture of swinging:

> The term hot wife refers to a married woman who has sex with men other than her spouse, with the husband's consent. In most cases the husbands take a vicarious pleasure in watching their wives' and the other male's enjoyment, or enjoy watching, hearing, or knowing about their wives' adventures. Husbands may also take part by engaging in threesomes, or arranging dates for their wives.[13]

Wikipedia goes on to identify a further subgrouping within hotwives: "A distinct subculture of wife-sharing, cuckolding, is a subgenre in which emphasis is placed upon the sexual humiliation of role reversal, with the woman free to flaunt her sexuality and show blatant enjoyment, and the husband restricted to a passive or subordinated role, possibly involving erotic sexual denial."[14]

Cuckolds separate themselves from the husbands of hotwives, in that cuckolds only have sex with their wives, at their wife's wish. Often, cuckold relationships involve the wife withholding sex from the husband, and even expressing how much they prefer having sex with their lover, to their husband. Cuckold relationships often involve themes of the wife ridiculing or humiliating the husband, which apparently earns her the title "humiliatrix." Much of the humiliation centers on the sexual inadequacies of the husband, notably in penis size or sexual ability, as compared to her lover(s). Cuckold relationships may involve forced, submissive bisexuality on the part of the husband and what is known as "creampies," where the cuckolded husband performs oral sex on his wife, after she has had unprotected sex with her lover, forced to consume her lover's semen from her vagina.

Suppressed (or repressed, take your pick) male bisexuality is a common interpretation of male fantasies of sharing their wives, with the idea that a man unable to fulfill his sexual attraction to another male might somehow fulfill this desire somewhat by the act of witnessing his wife having sex with another man.

Online, a husband described how he had invited his best friend to share his wife, with the specific intent of reinitiating a previous bisexual relationship he had had with his friend:

> I guess the idea of "sharing" my wife with him was somewhat my way of "using" her to be with him. She's kind of a "cold fish" sexually, and I like the idea of seeing her use her wares on another guy—especially a guy I trust and want to be close to sexually as well. I've recently admitted to him my bi-curiosity, and he let me stroke him and promised he'd stroke me back sometime. I want to suck him; however, he's not sure he'll return that favor. We've had more fun with each other since getting my wife involved.[15]

Some in polyamory report that their external relationships sometimes have little, if anything to do with sexuality. Many of their relationships are undertaken to meet emotional needs, rather than a desire for sexual adventure. Other polyamorists report that their choices are driven by the excitement and energy they get from new relationships, and from the intellectual and emotional stimulation of multiple partners. Initial research with polyamorists supports these anecdotal reports, with reported reasons for participation in polyamory including a need for both sexual and romantic variety, as well as commitment to personal growth and honesty, and needs that are not met in a single relationship. Although women identified "falling in love" as a reason for polyamory, it was consistently reported as a less important factor by most polyamorists responding to an online survey conducted in 2001. Personal development factors such as honesty to self, commitment to personal growth, and freedom were endorsed as driving reasons for polyamory more frequently than social values or reasons involving the needs of others.

The belief that women in nonmonogamous relationships are being taken advantage of relies upon the implicit assumption that it is actually the men, and only the men, that want sex outside the marriage, and that nonmonogamy is solely about the needs of the male. While little empirical research has examined the demographics and roles in polyamory, women are quite strongly represented in polyamorous literature. Female authors wrote most of the popular books about polyamory: *The Ethical Slut* by Easton and Liszt; *Polyamory, the New Love without Limits* by Deborah Anapol; *Redefining our Relationships* by Wendy O'Matik. *Loving More*, a monthly periodical dedicated to polyamory, is edited by a woman. Further, nonmonogamous relationships are present among the gay, bisexual, and lesbian communities, with significant attention offered over recent years to lesbian polyamory. As the approach of polyamory is more focused upon concepts of love and relationships, with less explicit attention to casual sexual encounters, it may be argued that polyamory is more "female friendly."

There has been no recent empirical research that examines the psychological or emotional functioning of those that are involved in polyamory, though some ethnographic and interview-based studies have indicated that women in polyamorous relationships typically report feeling empowered in their relationships with regards to their freedom, though they felt stigmatized by society's rejection of their relationship choices. Some limited studies were conducted in the late 1970s and early 1980s with individuals in sexually open marriages. The findings indicated little evidence of psychological dysfunction, and suggested that the personality types of these people tended toward nonconforming, unconventional creative achievers who enjoyed mental and social stimulation with secure self-image and ego.

Some of the writers and researchers who have examined the practice of swinging, notably Terry Gould, have described the degree to which women gradually take charge of a couple's swinging activity. They have explained that swinging, almost exclusively heterosexual, aside from the highly supported female bisexuality, is all about the female's sexuality, and male desire to share and experience it. As a result, the female holds the reins over it, and, in swinging, has control of the thing that everybody else wants. The hotwife/cuckold lifestyle seems to be an extension of that trend, wherein the question of whether or not the husband has sexual freedom with other women is of secondary importance, if it's an issue at all.

A typical characterization of swingers and open marriages paints these individuals as hippies, who just cannot seem to accept that the era of free love has ended. This seems a different flavor of the marginalization and deviancy theories, that those with extremely liberal views of sexuality and marriage must also have liberal beliefs and values about the rest of their lives. This is one area where consistent research has demonstrated opposite findings, at least with regards to swingers. Multiple studies conducted over the past few decades with swingers have indicated that they tend for the most part to identify more conservatively, and typically to vote Republican. In one study, 73 percent of swingers considered their political views moderate or conservative. Political research has shown that people tend to vote with their social class. Most swingers have above average incomes, and higher than average levels of education. Most swingers work in professional and/or management positions.

However, these higher-income, management-level, conservative swingers do have liberal views about sexuality, divorce, gender roles, homosexuality, and abortion, giving lie to the belief that if one has liberal views about sexuality, then they must be liberal about everything. One swinger interviewed by this writer described that he was usually not able to discuss his political views at swing parties, his stance was so at odds with the prevailing conservativism at such events, held in conservative Oklahoma. He joked that they probably schedule swing parties to coincide with the Republican caucus conventions, though as a liberal Democratic lawyer, that was one party to which he wouldn't be invited.

Swingers are heavily oriented towards heterosexual activity, though bisexual activity among women is prevalent and encouraged. Bisexual activity amongst men is almost unheard of among swingers, though some swing clubs have recently begun to hold events where bisexual male activity is accepted, and some swingers admit that behind closed doors, bisexual male activity has occurred amongst swingers. Many writers in the swinging community have stated that the antagonism to male bisexuality was a response to the AIDS crisis, and an effort to preserve swinging while limiting exposure to the disease.

Individuals living as swingers or in polyamorous lifestyles do have liberal views about sexuality, gender roles, and relationships. However, swingers do not appear to be liberal as a group, with regards to their political and social views, though they are less religious than the general American population. In contrast, preliminary research suggests that those who identify as polyamorous tend to be politically and socially liberal as a group, and are involved in nontraditional religion and spirituality much more than both swingers and the average American. At least with regards to those involved in polyamory as opposed to swinging, the social perception of the nonmonogamous as "hippies" may in fact be based in some reality. Whether such differences can be used to statistically distinguish swingers from polyamorists, or play a role in the development of swinging and polyamory, remains to be investigated.

Swingers are involved in swinging primarily for the sexual adventures. Research with swingers shows consistently that sexual variety, the thrill of forbidden sexual encounters and exhibitionism and voyeurism are the primary motivations reported by people involved in swinging. However, the third reason given by most swingers for their participation is making new friends and interacting socially with others who share their values and interests. Swingers express that they enjoy meeting people with whom they don't have to pretend monogamy. During the sexual adventures of swinging, ethical principles and respect for others are critical to participation in the lifestyle. "No" is the most powerful word in swinging, and those who cannot respect another's decision are excluded and even sometimes ejected from swing clubs. "No" is taken to a different level in many polyamorous relationships, with a common agreement around "veto power" giving some individuals the power to say "no," and end or prevent their primary partner's external relationship. In contrast to the "generalization" perception that the lives of swingers are entirely deviant, swingers have similar values to many nonswingers, valuing personal development over more social values. Research where swingers were asked to order their personal values in order of priority, having an "exciting life" was only ranked in tenth place, while self-respect, family security, and inner harmony were ranked first through third, respectively.

Like the authors of *The Ethical Slut*, swingers have embraced the term slut, with women encouraged to act and dress provocatively, in ways they've "always wanted to, but been afraid of." They attend swing parties dressed sexually and "slutty," and are rewarded with attention, even participating in contests where they show off, encouraged to behave in sexually provocative ways that can include real and simulated sex, all to the cheers and applause of their audience. Many such clubs have stages with poles, where the swingers can put on striptease shows and "pole-dances." The term "hedonism" has been co-opted as well, with popular sex-based resorts in Jamaica capitalizing on the name, attracting swingers, nudists, and exhibitionists to indulge their desires for hedonism.

Despite the perception of nonmonogamous relationships as unhealthy in one way or another, and ultimately doomed to failure, research shows that most people that have established nonmonogamous arrangements within their relationships are at least as satisfied as people in monogamous relationships. People in nonmonogamous relationships often report they are more satisfied and pleased with their relationship than they believe other couples to be, though this may result from their own history of dissatisfaction and divorce in prior relationships where they attempted monogamy. There are certainly individuals and couples that end up dissatisfied with attempts at negotiated nonmonogamy, and nonmonogamous relationships that have ended, whether or not nonmonogamy was a cause for the relationship's dissolution. For many individuals, couples, and families, nonmonogamy appears to be a positive component of their relationship, though there is little research that looks at nonmonogamy in the "lifetime" of relationships, at the general effects of nonmonogamy upon children and the family in general, or in comparison to monogamous relationships. Rates of mental illness, sexual abuse, and sexual dysfunction do not appear to be any more prevalent among those who have negotiated nonmonogamy than among the general population, or among those who have had extramarital affairs. In fact, findings suggest that couples who have established boundaries around nonmonogamy may experience more positive relationships than couples where infidelity occurs, and may communicate more frequently about personal and sexual needs than the typical couple with an agreement of monogamy.

Based upon the research and findings that do exist, it appears likely that the perception of such relationships as dysfunctional or doomed to failure is based more upon bias against nonmonogamy and cultural expectations about relationships, than upon the true effects of nonmonogamy. Despite predictions about the decline of swinging and other forms of nonmonogamous relationships, they have not disappeared. However, neither have they become widely accepted throughout Western culture. It appears likely that serial monogamy and covert infidelity will remain far more prevalent. Swinging and polyamory are not for everyone, and many, if not most, couples are not suited for such arrangements. However, for some couples and individuals, nontraditional relationships with different arrangements around monogamy serve as an alternative, despite the continuing legal and social restrictions against relationships that do not fit the monogamous couple held up as the cultural ideal.

It cannot be definitively stated whether those involved in non-monogamous relationships are psychologically and emotionally healthy, or whether a history of sexual trauma may predispose an individual to sexually nonmonogamous relationships. Many therapists seem to believe this is the case, but there is very little research to support or disprove it. What research has been done is dated or limited by research problems, but does seem to indicate that people in nonmonogamous relationships may tend to certain high-energy personality types. There is no evidence that suggests that they experience emotional or mental illness at rates higher than is present in the general population. There appears to be as much range in personality types and emotional and relationship functioning in these relationships as exists in the average individual, with no evidence to support the belief that poor mental health or dysfunction is driving participation in nonmonogamous lifestyles. Research with women in swinging relationships indicates that they seem to be as happy and satisfied in their sexual activities and lives as men, and are not presented as a group that has been sexually enslaved by men. In fact, as nonmonogamous relationships evolve, some relationship forms are dedicated to an explicit focus on women's needs. The perception of misogyny seems to be more focused upon the swinging lifestyle, rather than polyamory, and there is scant information about the experiences of polyamory. However, given the strong leadership that women have taken in defining the polyamory community, it seems unlikely that women are being universally victimized by polyamorous lifestyles. Whether or not such lifestyles are healthy remains a separate issue.

The question of whether or not human beings are naturally monogamous has little bearing on human behavior. Humans are naturally omnivorous, yet many people happily live exclusively on vegetarian diets. People can choose to be monogamous or not, but the research shows that a huge number of people do not choose monogamy, and have extramarital or extrapartner sexual encounters. The most common approach currently is serial monogamy, wherein individuals espouse monogamy so long as they are in a relationship, but move on to relationships with others once this relationship ends, often due to infidelity, as indicated in divorce literature. Some couples negotiate different boundaries around sexual and emotional fidelity, allowing, even encouraging, their partners to have relationships of one sort or another outside their own relationship. Despite the stigma associated with these types of relationships, there is no higher incidence of sexually transmitted disease, no evidence that individuals in such couples are emotionally or sexually disturbed, nor evidence that such out-of-the-norm sexual behavior is detrimental to the relationship. In fact, evidence suggests that such relationships have equivalent or slightly greater longevity compared to supposedly monogamous relationships where infidelity is the most frequent reason for separation.

These are not lifestyles or relationships that are suited for everyone, or for which every couple is suited. The O'Neills' attempt to foster the widespread development of open marriages to combat rising divorce rates was clearly unsuccessful, at least on that front. It seems likely that sexually open relationships will remain only a small percentage. The stigma against them remains strong, at least in the United States, despite the growing attention such relationships are receiving. Some polyamorists now claim, "we're the new gays," and champion gay marriage rights, hoping that legal recognition of their own relationships may come next. While swingers are persecuted and prosecuted in Arizona, similar attacks in San Diego ended in favor of constitutional arguments supporting privacy and free speech, with at least one swing club operator receiving a large financial settlement. In our neighbor to the north, the Canadian Supreme Court ruled in favor of swingers in 2005, finding that group sex among consenting adults is not a form of prostitution, or a threat to society. Despite the reactive fears of some vocal groups, it does seem that marriage as an institution can successfully survive alternate forms, and that there may in fact be some social benefits to the inclusion of those for whom traditional marriage is not a "good fit."

It remains to be seen whether social or legal recognition will come to those whose relationships are outside the established mold of heterosexual monogamous marriage. It seems likely that as homosexuals acquire the right to marriage or civil union in more states, the option of nonmonogamy may acquire more social acceptance and recognition, given the higher prevalence of such arrangements among homosexual and bisexual relationships. Because such relationships vary person to person and relationship to relationship, dependent upon the needs and desires of those involved, it does not seem likely that a single form of nonmonogamy will ultimately triumph, acquiring social and legal acceptance.

Instead, it is possible that the social view of intimate relationship may become more flexible, allowing relationships to flex to meet the needs of each individual. Such changes have already occurred in past decades, around gender roles within marriage, and the ability of women to work outside the home. As the needs and worth of the individual grow, in contrast to the overriding importance of the group, the next fifty years may bring more acceptance for those who find that the standard formulation of marriage and intimate relationship does not meet their individual needs.

MICHAEL AND JANICE

For the grass to be greener on the other side of the fence, there has to be a fence. Otherwise, it's all just grass.

Michael and Janice were fifty-five and fifty-two, both fit and attractive. Michael gave forth an extremely patient and gentle personality. His speech was educated and literate, and he came across as a very forthright and genuine individual with nothing to hide. He was the first individual I interviewed for this book who said that the promised confidentiality was irrelevant, that everyone in his life was aware of the nature of their marriage, and that he had nothing to hide.

Janice was an intense woman with an extremely direct gaze in her deep brown eyes. She was dressed conservatively, carrying a large purse with a large hardback book poking out of the top. Janice was very forthright, using blunt and direct language, but was surprisingly concerned about ensuring that she answered my questions. Throughout the interview, she would pause to ask whether her response was the answer I sought. When her husband described that he felt no real need for confidentiality, Janice visibly flinched, but said nothing. Janice was reserved at first, but as she warmed to the interview and grew more comfortable, a bright and full smile emerged.

The couple both identify as strongly liberal and Democrat, commenting that they tend to think, "Rush Limbaugh is the devil incarnate." Michael is very nonreligious, and Janice participates in an Eastern meditation school of thought. They say they're both worried about our country, and the environment, and people "using God's name to kill each other."

Michael was first to describe himself, and his upbringing. Janice remained reserved for some time, seeming to allow her husband to test the waters. Michael grew up in California, and has been married three times.

He and Janice have been married for fourteen years, and together for fifteen. Michael has two grown children, from previous marriages.

Janice said that she was not really "like most people." She was the youngest of six kids and grew up in a very wealthy and politically connected family. Janice and her siblings were abused as children, and Janice fled home when she was twelve. She literally ran away from home with a small circus and stayed with them for around six months, working carnival booths, and helping the elephant trainer. When the circus came back to town, Janice called an older sister, who notified the police. While Janice was gone, the children had been taken into state custody, and her father prosecuted for abuse. Janice lived in foster care until she was seventeen, when she left again, and went to college.

"It was hard for me to understand relationships, with people. It was very confusing to me. I started in therapy when I was eighteen, to try to begin to understand what reality was, and make sense out of what had happened. Because I was very confused, by the time I started college. In many ways I didn't have that strong social upbringing that said this is how you should be, and act, as a woman, so I was kind of making it up as I went along. I've never had a whole lot of rules, rules that said this is how you're supposed to act in a relationship, or this is how you're supposed to act with men. And so, it's been a process of me trying to figure it out. This is my only marriage. I really never thought I would ever get married, until I met Michael. I had a response in my body that said 'I'm going to marry this guy.' It's hard to explain. Moments after meeting him, I felt this tremendous shift in my body. I was thirty-six, and my whole way of thinking changed. We met when I was doing a Navajo Sundance, in Southern California. And he happened to be there too, I saw him, across a field. And I just kind of fell in love with him, right then and there."

Michael has had a "nontraditional" point of view of life since he was fifteen, and read books by Robert Heinlein and Robert Rimmer, both authors who described new, different kinds of sexual relationships. "When I met my first girlfriend, that was my frame. And one of our first conversations as we were getting to know one another was about this whole idea, and we really thought that a future life might be very interesting if we formed it with a third person, maybe a fourth person, involved in a mutually combined relationship. So that was one of the premises of our early relationship, was that we would live together for the rest of our life, and we would go find ourselves a wife, and maybe a husband or two. And, when we split up, and I met the woman who was to be my first wife, I said, 'Well, here's my idea,' and she said 'Not with me you're not; that isn't going to happen.' So I thought okay, maybe that was a childhood fantasy. I'm now ready to be an adult and have two kids and live a normal life under the conventional structure. And we did. We were monogamous; we played by the social rules of relationship, but ended the relationship, when she had an affair. She came home, said she felt guilty for having an affair, and maybe I was right, maybe there really isn't anything wrong with having other relationships. So she thought I should feel free to do that, and have a relationship, so I did. And she got jealous, couldn't handle it, and said okay, our marriage is over.

"So, when I met the woman who was to be my second wife, I had just a few years earlier been through the end of this marriage over issues of monogamy, and she said 'Not with me you're not having a nonmonogamous relationship,' and I said okay. And two years later or so, I came home and she was crying. She said she was pregnant, she'd been [having sex with] this other guy and got pregnant, and she was really sorry, it was a mistake."

Janice interjected, "Michael said, 'let's keep the child.'"

"Yeah, I said if you wanted to go and have unprotected sex with somebody so bad, and wanted to take a chance, you must really want a child, and if that's what you want, we'll keep the child. And she said no, she wouldn't do that, even though she wanted a baby. She went on to have more affairs, and eventually took off with some other guy. I was monogamous the whole relationship. Even though I wanted to have an open relationship, I wasn't going to do it in a sneaky way, it was going to be an arrangement. And then she came home one day and said she'd met this guy, and they'd been having great sex, and she was moving in with him. And I said you don't have to leave, just have great sex with him, that's okay.

"She said she couldn't do that, and moved in with him, and then I met Janice, and said, Okay, new rules. I'm not going to do this three times. I said to her, with great trepidation. 'What do you think of monogamy?' and she said, something to the effect of that she'd never successfully been monogamous. So one of the premises of our relationship was, that if we met someone that we were attracted to, that we would talk to the other person about it, really, pretty much get consent to explore the relationship.

Just having friendship doesn't take consent, but when it starts to move into a more intimate place, in order to create safety, we agreed that we would give the other person veto power."

Janice and Michael explained that they each have an agreement to "veto" activities by the other, and that in their agreement, no explanation or defenses are needed. They use this tool throughout their marriage, in their businesses and their life, beyond just their sexual relationships.

Though they agreed to be nonmonogamous in their marriage, they both agreed that they had to start by building their relationship with each other, and wouldn't start relationships with other people until they were ready. It was about a year before Michael said he was ready for Janice to pursue relationships with other men, it was about five years before Janice thought she was ready for Michael to do so.

Michael had the first emotional relationship with another person, but Janice had the first sexual relationships. It took a long while for Janice to open up about it, but eventually, she explained that for me to understand her, and her marriage to Michael, I had to know something about her that she rarely told other people.

Starting around age twenty-five, Janice became a prostitute. She was first a well-paid mistress to five businessmen, who paid for Janice to live in an apartment in Chicago, where she was visited by her lovers. She would spend three to five days with them, and they paid her cash. Janice did that for two years, saving her money, and then bought a salon. At age thirty-two, living in California, Janice went back to prostitution, as a massage therapist who offered erotic massage, and sometimes sex, to male customers. "I was doing massage, and started doing what's called sensual massage, where you give a guy a massage, and then a handjob at the end. Some men would approach me to do full service with them, and if I wanted to do full service with them, I would say okay, I'll do that with you. And it was a thousand dollars for two hours." This is how she was supporting herself when she met Michael, who quickly figured out what she was doing, but didn't ask her to stop. She had few relationships with men before Michael, most of whom "freaked out" when she told them about her profession.

Given Janice's concern about disclosing this history, and her early concerns about telling me what I "want to hear," I was careful in my response to her story. I told her that I appreciated her sharing this, but that I felt it was only relevant to her "story" if she herself felt it was. Inwardly, I'll admit that I was cringing. This woman had already disclosed a history of childhood abuse, and now a history of prostitution. In addition, she had shared that prior to Michael, she had never really had an intimate relationship that was supportive, or "healthy," by whatever definition one might choose. There was a lot of pain and rejection in Janice's life.

Men came to Janice, looking for someone to show them tenderness and kindness. Janice was good at what she did, and many men wanted her to become their mistress. Finally, Janice told one man that she would be, but only if he met Michael, and Michael agreed. The man was floored, but later invited Michael and Janice to a 49ers football game with him. The man became a close friend, and eventually business partner with Michael. Janice never became his mistress, and eventually their sexual relationship ended, replaced by their business friendship.

Janice continued to work as a prostitute for ten years after meeting—and marrying—Michael. They came to realize that it wasn't a matter of money for Janice, but about her self-worth, which was tied up in the "responsiveness of men to her," and her need for completely reliable independence, and a desire to "never be at anybody's mercy." But, after ten years working as a married prostitute, Janice finally stopped one day, when Michael went away on business. When he came back, she told him that she had quit. Removing this support from her life had dramatic consequences; Janice's health declined dramatically, and she spent the next four months in bed, being cared for by Michael.

Michael was never bothered by Janice's having sexual relationships with other men, and viewed these encounters as merely experiences, whether or not there was money involved. It was more difficult, though, when Janice stopped being a prostitute, and began having boyfriends, with whom she had emotional, and physical, relationships. Michael said that he does experience jealousy, but feels that jealousy in and of itself isn't a bad thing, but is just a thing, like being hungry or thirsty, or in pain because your foot hurts. Michael found that he could accept his wife being with other men, and come home "glowing" from her experience. He sometimes feels a "little churning" in his stomach, and some loss, but decided that he would instead take that energy, that experience, and work to make his wife enjoy coming home, so that she would always remember how good it was to come home to him. Only once did Michael tell

Janice that he had to "veto" her relationship, when he felt that it was becoming more important to Janice than their own relationship was.

Janice's boyfriends tend to be men who are different from Michael, and offer her qualities that Michael doesn't have. Most of the men have known Michael, but few became friends with him. Most had "resistance" to getting to know Michael, and some felt that if he really loved her, he wouldn't allow her to have relationships with other men. At least one man tried to entice Janice away from Michael.

But, these men couldn't have given Janice what Michael did. The ones who tried to steal Janice away believed that their relationship was one of deception and cheating, never understanding that for Janice, her relationships outside her marriage were not about cheating. "I never had rules really given to me. I lived my whole life doing what I wanted to do, doing it with whom I wanted, when it was appropriate. And, which meant I wasn't faithful. I never lied about that, I was never in relationships where I agreed to be monogamous. I don't lie, or like to lie. I don't sneak around."

Janice and Michael talk about everything, and are intensely committed to "telling their truth" to each other. They fight, but have found that they are better together in their marriage than they ever were apart. Both of them struggle with fears of abandonment in their marriage, triggered when they fight. When they fight, Michael has difficulty disengaging enough to allow the argument to subside, for fear of what the disengagement might mean. Janice reacts the opposite way and feels panicked and trapped when unable to back away from an argument. But, the couple has learned, through years of communication, "telling their truths," and therapy, how to balance their competing needs and fears, and to maintain their relationship with each other, even as Janice pursued relationships with other men.

"I've had experiences with a lot of men," said Janice. "I don't think I could do what we're doing with our relationship if I didn't love Michael the way I do, and if it wasn't absolutely clear to me that Michael is number one. That's the agreement I've made. It's a very important distinction to make. That is the distinction I've made in this relationship. No one will ever be more important for me than Michael is. I make that clear to everyone. Michael has been there for me, like no one else."

Janice and Michael have struggled, like many married couples, and admit that they've thought about divorce at times, but always fought through, in order to "stay engaged with each other." For them, staying engaged is the real "jewel in life," and the way to achieve the "beauty that comes from depth and intimacy."

Early on in their relationship, Janice suggested starting couple's therapy together, in order to "keep anything from going wrong." The couple spent a lot of time in therapy, together and as individuals. Their therapist thinks they're "the only couple he's ever known, who were able to do this lifestyle, and do it well," but he didn't assume that their nonmonogamy was the reason for them having problems. He didn't condone their lifestyle, or condemn it, but would instead work with them to succeed in their difficult choices.

"Most relationships start to die when a couple makes an agreement to ignore each other's issues. The life in a marriage comes from calling each other, from growing," agreed Janice. "And the minute you bring a third or fourth party into the mix, there's no hiding anymore. You're out there. I've never met anyone I respect and love more than I do Michael. So, it's not about seeking something that's missing, in a way. It's about added fun and enjoyment. It keeps our sex more alive, because it's not the same, it's broken up, variety in between. I think that's one of the reasons why sex is just off the charts for us."

"It's very good. You've probably heard the expression, for the grass to be greener on the other side of the fence," Michael paused, and there was the hint of a practiced routine with his wife, as she responded and filled his pause.

"There has to be a fence . . ."

Michael picked back up, "If there's no fence, it's just more grass."

For Michael and Janice, there is a lot of grass to explore. Janice says that this is the first relationship she's ever had where she wasn't bored after a year. Last month, she spent a weekend with another man, who she won't see again, because of the distance involved, but says that she had a blast with him. She doesn't have any boyfriends right now, but has men hitting on her constantly, from mechanics to neighbors. She told a recent story about her car breaking down, and her gardener kissing her, as he drove her to the dealership. Janice said she had to work hard to "make it safe for him to come back. I want him as a gardener, not as a lover."

Janice has done the "no-strings-attached thing. It's not a part of our relationship, not now, but it has been. I have enjoyed all my life meeting men, and if I wanted to just [have sex with] them, I did. I do that still. Very safely, I've never had any diseases. I've always had protected sex. The way we do it now, it's different, it's about relationships."

Two months ago, the couple had their one-and-only threesome with a guy. Janice was with a guy, and he invited her to call Michael and ask him to join them in bed. That was the first time the couple had sex together with another man. There have been times when Janice had sex with a lover while Michael was laying in the bed with them, and other times, when Janice had a lover stay over, and Michael slept in another bedroom. Michael is straight, but says that he's found that he "likes playing with guys. I can't quite imagine going on a date with a guy and getting in bed and making love, but if there's a woman there, and that's part of the picture, sure. That's cool. I've done that quite a few times."

Janice identifies as very heterosexual, and says that she feels comfortable coming back to Michael after being with another man. "Because of what I did, for ten years during our marriage. I'd see four men during the day, and then him at night and make love with Michael that night. I wasn't having sex with all four of those men though, I was having sexual experiences with them. He's the most nonjealous man I've ever been around in my life. And he enjoys hearing about it, when I've been with another man. It turns him on, my enjoyment with someone else."

"For the future, I still fantasize about, dream about, the possibility of us finding someone we would both like to share our life with," Michael said. "Emotionally and physically and sexually, cooking, just living. Twenty years ago, I'd have said that person would need to be a woman, in part because I'm heterosexual, and in part because of the chemistries between men and women makes me believe that having two people with projective energy and one woman trying to absorb it could be a little intense. But I'm more open to that possibility now—the possibility that the dream could be filled by some guy. But in my point of view, that would have to be a unique, special guy. More unlikely to find a guy where that chemistry works than a woman. But I still would like for that to happen."

"I'm just open to whatever comes our way. I don't feel it's something I have to search to find. If it happens, it happens. The way I see our lives going, we just bought our second house, probably going to buy a third one. We're investing, working in our businesses. We're very busy people. I don't think about how to plan our future, it's just being present to what is here right now. There's a lot on our plate right now," said Janice. "We have an unusual lifestyle. But the love I feel with Michael is so rich and deep; this is just one aspect of it. Michael's the finest person I've ever known in my life. I'm just really lucky to be in this relationship, and to have the freedom, and the trust that we have for each other. The fun parts of life are great and everything, but it's the hard times, and how we get through them together that brings such richness and joy and magic to my life and our relationship. I'm very grateful for that, and all the growing I've done because of the honesty we've had with each other and those difficult times, we've gotten through. In our relationship, we are free to be ourselves."

Michael agreed, "Even when we've been in phases where we agreed to not be with other people, or just haven't been with other people, the fact that it's a possibility and that the door is open, is such a huge decompression for me. I don't have to change anything now, there's no hole that needs to be filled, or hunger that needs satisfying. I'm so full, I have surplus."

Like other couples I've interviewed, Michael and Janice exemplify a deep, well-practiced level of communication within their relationship. A compelling component to their relationship was the intense, instantaneous bond they found in each other, and how the possibility of a nonmonogamous relationship was such a critical part of their bond and connection to each other.

In contrast to the belief shared by many, including therapists, that such a relationship would be likely to exacerbate and worsen any underlying emotional and childhood problems, the nontraditional relationship shared by Michael and Janice was incredibly healing to both of them. Both were able to work through and acknowledge many of the wounds they carried, and were able to seek solace and comfort from each other, as well as others. Having worked with many individuals who struggle in relationships, as they deal with the scars of childhood abuse, I found it intensely moving how Janice was finally able to allow someone to get emotionally close to her, and to be dependent on another person. Michael's undaunted patience and commitment to his wife was perhaps the only salve that could have ever helped her to heal the damage done in an abusive childhood.

Many who apply current psychological thinking to nonmonogamous relationships have assumed that a childhood of emotional or sexual abuse is implicitly involved in the development of such relationships. They assume that such individuals are unwilling or unable to have normal, "healthy" intimate relationships. And, they assume that the resistance to monogamy contributes to, and emerges from, the pathological emotional damage within the person. One could easily make the argument that Janice's early relationship problems, her difficulty just "understanding people and their rules," her "problems with monogamy" and her involvement in prostitution were all reflections of problems in emotional development. But, it seems unlikely that Janice could have ever been able to heal those wounds, and develop the trust and security she has, in a relationship bounded by traditional monogamy. Indeed, it seems likely that any such relationship, regardless of the partner, would have been doomed to the failure of other past relationships, where Janice pushed them away rather than allow herself to trust and depend on one person. It was only Michael's willingness to share his wife with other men that finally allowed her to trust him enough to share her heart and life with him.

Research has shown that most women fantasize about sexual situations in which they do not have to worry about the needs of their partner, and often, where they are receiving attention from their lover. In contrast, most men fantasize about situations where they are giving intense sexual pleasure and orgasm to a woman. The pleasure that Michael has, as his wife enjoys sex with another man, may be an extension of this phenomenon. Many husbands I interviewed described similar feelings, and explained their desires to watch their wives with other men, saying that they prefer to watch their wives' faces during the sex. If all they wanted was to see was genitalia and sexual intercourse, they'd watch pornography. "What is important to me is to watch the face of the woman I love enjoying herself."[1]

5

INSATIABLE WIVES THROUGHOUT HISTORY

Sex pleasure in woman is a kind of magic spell; it demands complete abandon; if words or movements oppose the magic of caresses, the spell is broken.

Simone de Beauvoir[1]

Betsy Prioleau, author of *Seductress: Women who Ravished the World and Their Lost Art of Love*, argues that as many as half of all women report difficulty achieving orgasm during intercourse, and that most women believe they themselves are less sexual than most other women. Prioleau suggests that the modern woman has lost the erotic power of femininity, giving up the sexual dynamism that by nature overshadows male sexuality. According to this New York professor of English literature, women are by nature polygamous, multiorgasmic, and able to handle a range and capacity of sexuality that men simply cannot match. Prioleau reviews the lives and history of hotwives and other seductresses since the dawn of time, celebrating the sexual dynamos that ravished men, often with their husbands' consent. Aphrodite (Venus to the Romans), whose legend emerged from the Sumerian and Babylonian goddess known as Inanna or Ishtar, cuckolded her husband Hephaestus (Vulcan). Zeus arranged the marriage of Aphrodite, hoping that Hephaestus could rein in the goddess's wildness. Hephaestus loved his wife and forged a magical girdle for her, which made her even more alluring and attractive to men. (No chastity belt here! This husband wanted men to be even more attracted to his wife, who really was a sex goddess.) For her treachery and infidelity with other gods, including Ares, she was at first imprisoned, but was freed, after the other gods witnessed her skills in bed with another god, Hermes.

Recorded history is replete with examples of wives and husbands who rejected monogamy for their wife. These were wives who embraced their sexuality with men other than their husbands, with, in most cases, the implicit or explicit consent of their husbands. Some of these husbands and wives experienced the social consequences of infidelity and cuckoldry, while others found their sexual exploits celebrated by society.

Tiberius was Roman Emperor in the decades during Christ's lifetime. To secure his throne, he married Julia, daughter of the previous Emperor Augustus. Julia was originally to marry the son of Marc Antony, who had Cleopatra as his mistress. Antony was defeated in his attempt at civil war, and so this marriage, pledged when Julia was only two years old, didn't happen. She did marry three times though. Her first husband died in war when she was sixteen, after only two years of marriage. Her second marriage lasted longer, around nine years, and Julia had four children. Her second husband, one of her father the emperor's favorite generals, also died in a military campaign. Finally, Julia married Tiberius, whom Augustus had chosen to succeed him. The marriage was strained, however, and the couple established some separation after about five years. Julia reportedly took lovers, which led to her ultimate downfall. Some historians, notably Seneca, have claimed that she prostituted herself, selling her "favors" in the Forum, though these claims are likely an exaggeration. In 2 BC, she received a letter from her father, divorcing her from Tiberius, and accusing her of plotting against the life of the emperor, as well as sexual infidelities with several men. Julia and several of her supposed lovers were exiled. One of her lovers committed suicide. Notably, this lover was a son of Marc Antony, and half-brother to her first betrothed. Julia eventually returned to Rome, but was imprisoned by her former husband, now emperor, who ordered she be isolated. Julia eventually died in her imprisonment, probably of malnutrition. Caligula, the famous sadistic, orgiastic emperor immortalized in history as a madman and murderer, was Julia's grandson.

Following the downfall of Caligula, Claudius took the throne as emperor of Rome. During the reign of Caligula, Claudius married his second cousin, Messalina. As accounted by Roman histories, including by the great historian Pliny, Messalina was simply too much for Claudius to handle. Stories of her sexual escapades abounded. Unsatisfied in the emperor's bed, Messalina reportedly snuck out at night, donning a blonde wig and servicing all comers in a brothel, where she "worked" under the name "Wolf Girl." According to the historian Juvenal, Messalina was usually the last "girl" to leave, after other prostitutes had left for the night, and she often left unsatisfied. She worked semi-anonymously, and charged no more than the going rate. When the brothels weren't enough, she sought sexual partners in taverns, sometimes dancing nude on tabletops, to entice men into her clutches. In one infamous episode, Messalina challenged Rome's leading prostitute to a battle of skills, as to which could satisfy more men in a day. Messalina won hands down, serving twenty-five men in a twenty-four-hour period. Messalina's downfall came though, when her somewhat oblivious husband was awakened to anger by Messalina's choice of a political competitor as sexual partner. Messalina, having fallen in love, both wed and bedded a young noble named Silius, consummating their relationship in bed before a crowd of onlookers. When Claudius learned of this, fear that Silius and Messalina might depose him triggered a response where stories of Messalina's promiscuity had not. Before dawn, both Silius and Messalina were dead.

In 1631, Mervyn, Lord of Castlehaven, was tried in England for crimes that included having his servants rape his wife in front of him. Mervyn then had sex with those male servants, both giving and receiving anal sex. Mervyn also had one of these servants attempt to impregnate his twelve-year-old daughter. The earl's wife reported to the court that on one of the first nights of their marriage, her husband called his male servants to their bedroom, ordering them to strip, and forcing his wife to look upon their bodies. He told his wife that if she slept with the men, it would be his fault, not her own. (Nice of him to take the blame, wasn't it?) On trial for his actions, Castlehaven defended himself, admitting that he had in fact slept with the servants, but that the other allegations were false, invented by his son, who desired the earl's title. His defense was notably unsuccessful, and the earl was duly removed of his head. His two male servants were also executed for their role in the rape of his wife. During later years, his wife was accused of being a lascivious woman, and her promiscuity was alleged to have been behind the earl's true downfall, through political manipulations she engineered through her lovers.[2]

One of the most infamous cuckolds in history was Roger Palmer, the British earl of Castlemaine. In 1659, he chose Barbara Villiers to be his wife, in a marriage destined for tragedy. While Palmer was a devout and studious Catholic, his wife Barbara was not. According to most histories, the only thing Barbara was devoted to seems to have been sexual encounters with any man who struck her fancy. A painting of Barbara, done by Sir Peter Lely, the most famous portrait painter in Britain of the day, shows a slender, dark-haired, and attractive woman. She bore six children throughout her marriage to Palmer, and it is believed that none of them were Palmer's. One daughter, Anne, had three different men, including Palmer, claim her as their daughter. Barbara became a mistress to Charles II, king of England, but was no more faithful to him than to Palmer. Barbara had numerous lovers amongst the London Court and intelligentsia, and her promiscuity was by no means secret. Palmer was ridiculed throughout London gossip as a cuckold, and his wife was labeled as a slut, royal harlot, and whore in writings of the day. By the British law of the day, Palmer could have divorced his wife, but her status as a favorite of the king promised that this would be a politically suicidal thing to do, and Palmer's devout Catholicism precluded divorce anyway. When James II succeeded Charles to the throne of England, Palmer was sent to the Vatican as an ambassador. However, his status as a cuckold preceded him to Rome, and was the likely reason for Palmer's abject failure as a statesman. He died after a political imprisonment, still married to Barbara, who wasted little time in marrying another man. Ironically, it turned out that he was already married to another woman, and this marriage quickly failed. Barbara followed her poor, humiliated husband into death, approximately four years later.

The Borgias were the family made famous by Niccolo Machiavelli, for their complex, vicious, and murderous politics. The father of the family, Rodrigo Borgia, was a powerful Italian who later became Pope Alexander VI. Lucrezia, his daughter, was married three times, and betrothed twice also, all marriages and arrangements that were driven by her father's politics. Stories of the Borgia's sexuality are almost as compelling as their predilection for murderous politics. According to papal records, Lucrezia's father hosted an orgy once, in which prizes were awarded to the men who had "carnal knowledge" of the greatest number of courtesans. Prizes were awarded by onlookers as judges, including Lucrezia.

Her first marriage was to Giovanni Sforza, in order to obtain the support of Giovanni's family. That support wasn't long needed and, according to legend, Lucrezia went to her husband and informed him that her father had directed her brother to murder Giovanni. Giovanni promptly fled, and some stories suggest that there was never a murder plot, merely a plot by Lucrezia to rid herself of an annoying husband. After much familial negotiation and debate, their marriage was annulled and Giovanni was paid off, though he had to agree that their marriage had not been consummated due to his impotence. Lucrezia was soon betrothed again, but not before she mysteriously delivered a baby. Her father issued two papal bulls about this male infant, later named Giovanni Borgia. Although the documents never publicly indicate that Lucrezia was the mother, the first bull indicates that the infant was conceived in an affair prior to her marriage to Sforza, and the second indicates that Pope Alexander VI (her father!) was the father of the child. This second bull was not made public, however, and most assumed that Giovanni Borgia was actually the child of Lucrezia and her brother, Cesare, who was a cardinal in the Church.

Lucrezia married again, but this time her brother Cesare actually did kill her husband, ostensibly due to both jealousy of his brother-in-law and political intrigue. Lucrezia's third and final marriage was to Alfonso d'Este, prince of Ferrara and a marriage arranged by her father yet again. Lucrezia was not long faithful to Alfonso, though she was reportedly quite fond of him. She soon entered into a love affair with Francesco Gonzaga, who was married to Alfonso's sister. Her affair with Francesco was long and heatedly sexual, ending only when Francesco contracted syphilis. Lucrezia also had a passionate love affair with the Italian poet and scholar Pietro Bembo, who had been hired by Alfonso. The love letters between she and Bembo were stored in a library at Milan, and were famously lauded by none other than Lord Byron (to whom we shall return shortly). Lucrezia died in 1519 from childbirth at the age of thirty-nine.

The Marquise du Chatelet, Gabrielle Émilie le Tonnelier de Breteuil, was born in Paris in 1706 and died a mere forty-three years later. But in her short life, this vivacious, brilliant woman led a life that fostered intellectual development. Married to a French governor and soldier, in 1725, Émilie entered a life of politics and intellectualism. While she bore three children to her husband, he was often away on political and military duties. Émilie began to take lovers, and was apparently drawn to men who could expand her mind. One lover was Pierre Maupertuis, a leading mathematician, who taught Émilie mathematics in a time when women were largely excluded from the sciences. With Pierre, Émilie began to pursue an entrance into the male halls of intellectual discourse. Excluded from some, by virtue of her sex, Émilie returned, dressed as a man, and forced her way in. Soon though, Émilie began a long relationship with one of the foremost authors and philosophers of the day, François-Marie Arouet, who famously took the pen name, Voltaire. Her relationship and love affair with Voltaire was to last for the next two decades, and to the end of her life.

Émilie did not forego her relationships with her other big-brained lovers, but Voltaire became her closest confidant. Her husband was aware of their relationship, and indeed, the three developed their own relationship when he returned from his duties, and the three occasionally shared a home together. Émilie published philosophical works, both in collaboration with Voltaire, and independently. Her most significant accomplishment appears to be her translation into French of Sir Isaac Newton's *Principia*. At age forty-three, Émilie died in childbirth, delivering the child of yet another lover, the poet Jean-François de Saint-Lambert. Voltaire, her husband, and Saint-Lambert were all present, though Émilie had apparently managed to enlist the help of Voltaire and Saint-Lambert in convincing her husband that the child was actually his.

Voltaire later described Émilie thus, in his preface to her translation of Newton's *Principia*:

No woman was ever more learned than she was, yet no one deserved less than she did to be called a blue-stocking. She only ever spoke about science to those from whom she thought she could learn; never did she discuss it to attract attention to herself. She was not ever seen gathering around her those circles which wage battles of the mind, where one sets up a kind of tribunal and passes judgment on one's century—which then in its turn judges you most severely. For a long time she moved in circles which did not know her worth and she paid no attention to such ignorance. . . . I saw her, one day, divide a nine-figure number by nine other figures, in her head, without any help, in the presence of a mathematician unable to keep up with her.[3]

In the 1800s, Leopold Ritter von Sacher-Masoch, after whom the term "masochism" was coined, may have been the first known figure to intentionally explore and pursue cuckoldry by his wife. His wife Aurora revealed in her autobiography that her husband had induced her to take on lovers, that he might experience the suffering brought on by infidelity.

Leopold was born in 1836, and grew up with a fascination of martyrdom, executions, and torture. As a prepubescent, he witnessed a female relative, a countess, who had taken a lover other than her husband. Surprised by the husband and two friends that accompanied him, the Countess flew into a rage and drove off the husband and his compatriots, lashing a whip at them as they fled in fear. The husband later returned, kneeling to his wife and begging her forgiveness.

Contrary to the image of a cuckold weakling, Leopold was no coward, despite the fantasies of subjugation and female domination that he began to explore. In 1848, at age thirteen, this son of a police officer stood guard at a barricade, and used pistols to defend his family and community amidst a political revolution.

As an adult, and an accomplished writer, Leopold was approached by Aurora Rümelin, who would later wed him. Aurora approached him under an air of seductive mystery, a mystery which enthralled Leopold. Aurora called herself Wanda, the name of one of Leopold's female characters, in order to intrigue and entice her future husband. They were married in 1873, and it wasn't long until Leopold had induced his young bride to issue him a daily whipping. Leopold began to beg his wife to take a lover, even posting an advertisement in a local newspaper that she sought an "energetic" young male companion (even then, the nineteenth-century version of Craigslist was the cuckold's best friend).[4] According to Aurora's autobiography, she did in fact meet a potential paramour at a tavern. But, when this gentleman learned the nature of their meeting, he chivalrously escorted her home safely and unsullied. It is noteworthy that Leopold's wife, while willing to flog and otherwise punish her submissive husband, was resistant to carry through on this demand. Despite Leopold's repeated pleadings, and his frequent machinations to arrange instances whereby his wife would be unfaithful, she fulfilled this desperate need of his only once, during a later encounter.

Indeed, it was this issue that ultimately led to her divorce of Sacher-Masoch. Both went on to remarry, though it is unclear how great a role Leopold's sexual fantasies played in his second marriage. In a fascinating intellectual extension of Leopold's desire for dominant, powerful women, he edited a literary magazine in the 1880s, which was one of the few that was then publishing articles arguing for women's rights and suffrage. Aurora later published an autobiographical tale of her ten-year marriage to Leopold, renewing her pen name of Wanda, in *The Confessions of Wanda von Sacher-Masoch*, which recounted the degree to which she felt compelled to meet her husband's desires, in order to maintain the safety of herself and their children.

Lilith, the wife whose story is told in interlude 6, was quite conversant in sadomasochism lore. She described Leopold's nagging pleadings to his wife as "topping from the bottom," where the submissive in a BDSM relationship assumes control of the relationship, scripting each action of the dominant to meet their own internal demands. In contrast, the "true submissive," gives up control to the dominant, who chooses whether or not, and which, of the submissive's needs to meet.

Alessandro Cagliostro was the pseudonym of an Italian occultist, called a fraud by many, whose real name was Giuseppe Balsamo. He traveled Europe in the last years of the eighteenth century, using his skills in chemistry, the history of the occult, forgery, and general flim-flammery, to swindle nobility of their riches. He married Lorenza Feliciana, at the age of fourteen, living with his young wife's parents for a time. That arrangement soon ended, as the parents were offended at the way young Balsamo induced his bride to display herself, wearing revealing clothes. The couple left, and Balsamo apprenticed himself to a master forger, who taught him how to use his skills at drawing to render false documents. Balsamo would later use these skills to great effect, even forging a letter for the great lover, Casanova, later in life. The price for this apprenticeship? Balsamo's teacher desired Lorenza in his bed, a fee both Balsamo and Lorenza were apparently happy to pay. Across their lives together, Lorenza served as Balsamo's assistant, as he took on the trappings of his role as Count Cagliostro.

At one point, she eloped with a male lover, Duplaisir. Cagliostro did not endorse this relationship, and put out charges against his wife, who was subsequently apprehended and imprisoned for several months, as punishment for her adultery. Despite her time in prison, their professional relationship continued, and soared as Cagliostro was initiated into the Masonic Rites, and championed an offshoot, based upon the mythology of Egypt. This Masonic tradition was heretical and condemned by the Scottish Rite of Masons, as Cagliostro admitted women as well as men. The rituals of the Egyptian Masons were overseen by Lorenza, in her role as "Grand Mistress." The rituals involved nudity, led by Lorenza, who disrobed in front of all initiates, male and female, inducing them to likewise cast off the mortal bonds of clothing. Whether or not the rituals also involved orgiastic sex, led by Lorenza, is a matter of some "heated" debate.

Following a complex scandal known as "the affair of the diamond necklace," wherein Cagliostro was accused and prosecuted for attempting to defraud French nobility (which he was, surprisingly in this case, innocent of), Cagliostro and his wife fled France for London, and then Rome. In Rome, Cagliostro was imprisoned by the Inquisition as a heretic. Though unconfirmed, rumors have persisted that Lorenza had proffered the charges against her husband, that led to his arrest. Sentenced to life in prison, Cagliostro died in an Italian prison, six years after his arrest. Lorenza was also arrested by the Inquisition, and also sentenced to life in prison as a heretic. She reportedly also died in prison, a year before her husband. Cagliostro, and his wife, are occult personages of some significant charm, who make regular appearances in vampire literature, where Lorenza is portrayed as an opponent of Dracula, and in comic books, where Cagliostro is sometimes described as an immortal with mystical powers.

At the age of seventeen, Jane Elizabeth Digby married a British lord, a marriage that was to last four years, and ended when she fled Britain for Europe, to bear the child of another man. Lord Ellenborough, her first husband, was described as an unattractive man, who was nevertheless quite wealthy and powerful. He desired a young beautiful wife who would bear him an heir. What he got instead led to his own humiliation and downfall. Left to her own devices in London, as her husband worked at politics, Jane's beauty drew much attention and many invitations to society events. She remained faithful for two years to her husband, but at last invited a young intellectual into her bed.

That young man, a museum researcher, later praised God for his graciousness at granting him such fortune, as to share the young wife's bed.

Jane then entered into another affair with a male cousin, a colonel in the British military. Her husband briefly woke himself from his work to remember that he wanted to have an heir, and would have to do something about it if he was to succeed in this wish. Jane did bear him a son, who died at the age of two. After the son's birth, Jane no longer took her husband into her bed, but found another lover, an Austrian prince. Prince Schwarzenberg was a dashing, handsome, and charismatic man whom Jane met at a government reception. Schwarzenberg was known to have a mesmerizing effect upon women, and Jane was not immune. They were soon lovers, and shortly after, the prince established lodgings quite near to the London home of Jane's parents. Jane found time to visit the prince each day. On at least one occasion, they left the drapes open as they romped in the prince's bed, and a neighbor described witnessing their encounter in explicit detail when called upon during later legal hearings. Jane's husband was informed of the growing public scandal, but refused to believe it of his young wife. At last, pregnant with the prince's child, Jane confronted her husband and informed him of her infidelity, her pregnancy, and her love for the prince. Jane and the prince fled to the Continent, and away from the scandal that continued to gain steam.

Despite the efforts of both Ellenborough and his political allies, the Parliamentary discussion of his bid for a legal divorce was neither short, nor genteel. Britain was hungry for details, and every neighbor, chambermaid, and servant who could offer details was called to testify. Jane had not been discreet, even when they did remember to close the drapes, and there were plenty of witnesses to describe Jane's sexual voraciousness, and her husband's neglectful passivity. The divorce was granted by the government, but Lord Ellenborough was disgraced as a man who had abandoned and neglected his beautiful wife. By letting her go to bed alone every night, he had let her hunger build until, starved, she engaged in the indiscreet behaviors that so captivated the country.

Jane and Schwarzenberg's relationship was not idyllic, and he soon left her, taking their infant daughter with him. In Paris, in the midst of the beginnings of the French Revolution, Jane developed a relationship with the French writer Honore de Balzac, who in turn immortalized her as the character of Lady Arabella Dudley, an aristocratic English nymphomaniac, in his tale *The Lily of the Valley*. Three other contemporary writers based characters on Jane, though all three were much less flattering towards her.

Jane continued her whirlwind of a romance-driven life. Captivated by her reputed beauty, King Ludwig I of Bavaria invited her to his kingdom, and soon took her into his bed as a lover. Jane became pregnant, and abruptly married a baron of Ludwig's court, bearing a child that was probably Ludwig's. Jane had two more children with her husband the baron, until she fell in love with a Greek count, Theotoky. She carried on yet another secret affair with the count, until her husband the baron learned of it, and catching them in the act, challenged the Greek count to a duel. The baron's hand was faster with his pistol, and the count wounded. Proclaiming his innocence to the baron, the count was carried to the home of Jane and her husband, where all three lived together as the count was nursed back to health. Jane at last confessed her love for the count, and the baron gave the couple his blessings, and Jane her freedom. Jane and the baron remained lifelong friends.

Five years later, after touring Europe extensively with Count Theotoky, Jane married him in Greece. They remained married ten years, and by all accounts, Jane was faithful to the count, but their love and connection simply ran out, dying with the accidental death of their only child. Within months of the end of their marriage, Jane had another lover: King Otto, the son of King Ludwig I, and king of Greece.

Jane soon tired of being the mistress and lover of this king as well, and traveled to Italy and the Mediterranean, where, most stories agree, her promiscuity and sexual desires were finally fully unleashed. Over the next few years, she had as many as six different husbands, and countless lovers, even at one period having three Italian lovers simultaneously. Finally, exhausted and dissatisfied, Jane fled to the deserts of Arabia. There, Jane's beauty and poise captivated a young sheik. When Jane calmly and expertly rode a horse that the sheik had deemed unbreakable, the sheik told Jane she could buy the horse, but only by sharing his bed. Jane demanded the sheik first send away his harem of three wives, asserting that she had no need to compete with other women. Overcome by desire for this woman whose assertiveness was so foreign to the sands of his land, the sheik sent away his wives and took Jane into his bed. Jane soon left Saleh the sheik, and continued her explorations of the desert land. She had other lovers, but at last, at the age of forty-eight, settled down with Medjuel al Ezrab, a Bedouin nobleman of substantial learning and education. They remained married for the rest of their lives, twenty-six years; by all accounts it was a very happy marriage for both of them. This is not to say though, that Jane's appetites or allure were diminished. At the age of seventy-three, Jane was still prompting her husband to make love to her more frequently, and at the age of seventy-one, a young man in his twenties tried unsuccessfully to seduce her. Jane Digby died in 1881, at the age of seventy-four.

Victoria Woodhull was the insatiable wife who could have been president of the United States. In 1872, Victoria Woodhull, former wife of Dr. Canning Woodhull, ran for president on a platform that included the celebration of free love, and every woman's right to experience orgasm. This former prostitute, spiritualist, and clairvoyant was born in frontier Ohio in squalid poverty. An intelligent child, she received only three years of formal schooling due to the family's hardships. At the age of fifteen, Victoria and her sisters formed a medicine show, and joined that cadre of scoundrels and hucksters that traveled the frontiers of America, peddling fake medicines and healings and putting on spiritualist shows. Victoria married her first husband, Canning Woodhull, a physician from New York, at the tender age of fifteen. But, this spirited young girl was soon holding the reins of their marriage, and it was all Canning could do to keep up. He followed his young bride to California, where she took briefly to the stage, before learning of the growing financial success of mediums, who held séances and spiritual ceremonies. Victoria and her family opened a business as fortunetellers and clairvoyants, where Victoria and her younger sister as often sold their bodies as they sold the future. Chased from their business for failing to pay police bribes as prostitutes, Victoria and family toured several states, taking their unique blend of sex and séance to a gullible and paying public. In St. Louis, a writer for the newspaper attempted to unveil Victoria as a fraud, but was seduced by her instead. She took this new lover, Colonel James Harvey Blood, in tow, cuckolding her acquiescent and now alcoholic husband, whom she kept around to care for their children. In Chicago, she accused Canning of infidelity, and divorced him, though he remained a part of her entourage.

Seeking publicity, Victoria and Blood caught upon the idea of her running for president. Seizing the fever of the growing suffrage movement to offer the vote to women, Victoria slowly gained some legitimate and credible support. Attacked by other women for her history as a prostitute, she was defended by Elizabeth Cady Stanton, who called upon women to stand united, and not attack one another, when men were the real enemy. The fact that Victoria kept two male lovers, both ostensibly her husband, fed the press into a frenzy. Victoria engaged in political wrestling matches, and some verbal ones as well, with Susan B. Anthony, but Susan eventually won, named as the presidential candidate by the Suffrage Association. Victoria created her own party, and secured a nomination, but the end of this chapter was near.

Victoria's presidential campaign died a quiet death, and she received few popular votes, though the fact that she had engineered even having her name on the ballot was an impressive feat. Victoria resumed her career as a spiritualist, and her love affairs with men continued. At thirty-five, she seduced a nineteen-year-old college student, who later told an interviewer that the end of their relationship came when Victoria told him that she was sending him into the bed of her younger sister. When young Benjamin Tucker refused, Victoria insisted that if he was to love her, he must also love her sister Tennessee. Victoria at last drove Colonel Blood away, when she suspected him of infidelity. Despite her many male lovers, and her support of free love, this was apparently a female-dominated road. She divorced Blood, complaining that she knew that he had consorted with a prostitute—not an untrue statement, in fact, given her own history.

Victoria eventually moved to London and married John Martin, an aristocratic businessman and banker, who undertook to protect his wife's name from the scandalous stories that filled the press concerning her past. The couple traveled to the United States often, filing libel and defamation suits, though few were won and those that were generated little satisfaction. In 1892, Victoria was again nominated for president, but lost again, winning not a single state. Victoria went on to embrace educational reform and used the wealth of her husband to support significant philanthropic endeavors. When she died in 1927, the press was gentle, describing her suffragist history, her political and philanthropic endeavors. The stories of free love, multiple husbands, prostitution, and the value of the female orgasm were left on the editing floor. The Woodhull Freedom Foundation and Federation is an organization founded in 2003, to champion the rights of sexual freedom as a basic and essential human right.

> I am a Free Lover. I have an inalienable, constitutional, and natural right to love whom I may, to love as long or as short a period as I can, to change that love every day if I please!

So after all I am a very promiscuous free lover. I want the love of you all, promiscuously.[5]

Violet Gordon Woodhouse, one of the greatest pianists of the early years of the twentieth century, lived for decades with not one, but four husbands. A child prodigy, known for playing the harpsichord, Violet was born in Britain in 1872, and died in 1951. In 1895, she married Gordon Woodhouse, though she apparently set limits on their marriage, that they would not share a bed, and would not have sex. Though she did love him, Violet went on to take many other lovers during their marriage. Three additional men moved in with them, and the family lived together for decades, referred to as the "Woodhouse circus." The expansion of her family began with Violet's relationship with British aristocrat Bill Barrington, the tenth Viscount Barrington. Two other men moved in within the next five years. Ultimately, the family, and their unique arrangement, was interrupted by World War I, and never returned to this polyamorous stability.

A fascinating cluster of sexually voracious wives swirled around the famous Romantic poet, Lord Byron. George Gordon Byron, sixth Baron Byron, known as Lord Byron, was a romantic poet and man of towering historical and literary stature. He also appears to have been something of a magnet for wives who could not, or would not, be monogamous. In his life, his confidantes and lovers included wives such as Elizabeth Milbanke, known as Lady Melbourne; Anna Louise Germaine Necker, known as Mademoiselle de Stael; Lady Caroline Lamb, known as Lady Oxford; Teresa Guiccioli; and Claire Clairmont. Of these women, only Claire was not married to another man.

Anna Louise Germaine Necker was not reported to be an attractive woman, and even once said that she would trade half her considerable wit to be more beautiful. Somewhat broad and coarse features belie the intelligence of this woman who stood up to Napoleon Bonaparte, and the sexuality that led her to have numerous lovers and affairs across the whole of Europe. Married at age twenty, Anna was born into an extremely wealthy Swiss family. Anna came by her seductive charms honestly; her mother had married Anna's wealthy father, after stealing him away from his lover at the time, the woman who employed Anna's mother as a servant. Anna's father used wealth to secure his son-in-law, Eric Magnus, the Baron de Stael-Holstein, an ambassador's position, but Anna was not taken with her husband, an arranged and unstimulating marriage. Early in her marriage, Madame de Stael embraced literature and began an accomplished literary career. Her most famous novel was *Corinne,* a romantic tale that Byron loved, as it celebrated those who were not virtuous. Byron called her a very clever woman, and wrote that "She thought like a man, but alas! She felt like a woman."[6]

In grief after the death of her first child, a daughter, Anna first pursued active and aggressive adultery, entering into sexual liaisons with several different men. Though not as beautiful as she may have wished to be, that sharp wit which she was willing to trade away was what drew men to her like flies to honey. Seeking lovers to soothe her grief set something of a lifelong precedent for her. She wrote once to a lover, explaining that she had taken yet another lover, so that she might gain "a sort of excitement that would relieve for a moment the terrible weight that was pressing on my heart."[7] In 1794, Madame de Stael met Benjamin Constant, an awkward, gawky, but well-educated man who was to become a star in French politics. Constant and she became lovers and remained so throughout their lives. She separated from her husband in 1797, after he demanded to no longer be cuckolded, though they remained legally married. Her relationship with Constant was not monogamous either, and he indulged her passions. Entranced by the rising flame of Napoleon, Anna wrote to him, attempting to establish a relationship, ostensibly to influence his politics, though she did attempt to bring him to her bed as well. Once, she even snuck into Napoleon's home, and cornered him alone in the bath, but to no avail. At last, she turned her pen and sharp wit against Napoleon's politics and began to gather intellectuals around her criticisms of Napoleon. Napoleon banished her from Paris.

Goethe described Anna, saying that "Her great ambition is to subjugate political men and to impress upon them the ascendancy of her opinions." At forty-five, Constant and Anna finally separated, as she refused to marry him. Anna took a twenty-three-year-old Italian lover, who she later married. Anna returned to Paris after Napoleon's defeat at Waterloo and returned to her intellectual pursuits. She died in 1817, having influenced ideas, politics, men, and nations throughout her life.

Though Napoleon rejected Anna de Stael, both his wife and his own sister followed in the adulterous, sexually promiscuous footsteps laid by de Stael and others. Napoleon himself was known as "Commander Cuckold" to his troops, due to Josephine's blatant relationship with Hippolyte Charles. Bonaparte's sister, Pauline, was a beauty who posed nude for the Italian sculptor Canova, who used her as a model for Venus, in a sculpture that showed the goddess reclining nude. Pauline had a beautiful body, and little if any reluctance to show it and share it with men whom she found attractive. Napoleon arranged her marriage at age sixteen to a young French general, hoping this would settle his sister down. The general died in Haiti six years later, at a political post assigned by Napoleon. Pauline mourned her husband, but celebrated her return to Paris by diving deep into the waiting pool of eligible men, and again Napoleon found a husband to contain his sister, or at least to give her a tinge of propriety. She married Prince Camillo Borghese, an extremely wealthy Italian, known for his diamonds, but not for his intellect. Unfortunately, the prince appears to have been impotent, and Pauline began to indulge herself with man after man, and was publicly compared to the sexually insatiable Messalina. Borghese separated from her, due to her blatant cuckoldry of him, though Pauline's brother would not allow a divorce.

Pauline then used the wealth at her hands to live a life of sybaritic excess, indulging her whims, and, in particular, her taste for men. Pauline had a male servant who carried her nude each morning to a bath of water and milk. Pauline would remain in her bath for hours and delighted in receiving male visitors there, that she could display the body she so celebrated. One famous affair with a painter actually appears to have challenged even her erotically supercharged body. Nicolas Philippe Auguste de Forbin was a talented but impoverished painter who Pauline hired as her chamberlain. But what Nicolas lacked in finances, he reportedly made up for in other forms of endowment. Pauline indulged herself with her lover for a year, but at last fell into a physical depression, which physicians diagnosed as the result of her lover's "gigantism," his ability to maintain an erection for long periods, and the "undue friction" that thus resulted from their lovemaking.[8] Pauline at last separated from her well-endowed lover, and her health returned.

Devoted to her brother, Pauline spent four months with him on the island of Elba during his imprisonment. At forty-five, Pauline died of cancer, and her last wish was to have her coffin closed, and the nude Canova statue displayed instead, that people might see her as she had truly been, beautiful, confident in her nudity and sexuality, exuding the passion and erotic power of the Goddess of Love.

Elizabeth Milbanke, a dark-eyed beauty descended from a wealthy Yorkshire family, married Sir Peniston Lamb at age seventeen, becoming Lady Melbourne. Lord Melbourne had a forty-year career in Parliament, a political career largely undistinguished and mostly forgotten. His wife however, cast a far bigger shadow. Bored by her husband, Elizabeth began entertaining eligible, influential males in her London home. Intelligent, conversationally eloquent, and beautiful, Elizabeth quickly became the center of much male attention. Her political and social influence was extended by her willingness to invite these eligible men into her bed. She had many powerful, wealthy, and noble lovers, and was even once "sold" by one lover to another for thirteen thousand pounds (an astonishing figure for early in the nineteenth century). Stories held that Elizabeth herself pocketed some of the proceeds of that sale.

Elizabeth advised powerful men, as to their choices in wives, and their politics. She was a mistress to the Prince of Wales, who became king as George IV, and "earned" her husband a promotion to the noble rank of viscount. Subsequently, her husband was ironically appointed to a formal court position, as lord of the bedchamber, a position where he assisted the king or Prince of Wales in dressing and guarded access to his chambers. Given that his wife was in bed with the prince at the time, one certainly wonders at this duty. The Lady Melbourne had six children, and the identities of their respective fathers remain, in many cases, a mystery. One of the male friends Elizabeth acquired later in life was Lord Byron, who certainly loved scandalous women. Byron later had an affair with the wife of Elizabeth's son William Lamb, an affair that Elizabeth played some advisory part in, assisting the poet in arranging his assignations with the lady's daughter-in-law. Byron later bemoaned the fact that Elizabeth was so much older than he, called her a "best friend," and said that if she had been a few years younger, he would have been a fool for her.

William Lamb, son of the infamous Lady Melbourne, courted Caroline Ponsonby for three years. A somewhat nervous, intense child, Caroline received no formal schooling, as she was judged too delicate for the rigors of schooling, and she lived a pampered, spoiled life as a child, though she later learned four languages on her own and embraced theater and music as her passions. But, after four years of marriage, Caroline fought her boredom by pursuing first intellectual pursuits with other intellectuals, and then began to pursue other men. Her husband was aware of her affairs, but indulged his wife, believing this would soon pass. But, Caroline Lamb then found a new source of excitement, in the young burning star that was Lord George Gordon Byron. Inflamed with his literary genius, she aggressively pursued the young poet, and lured him into her bed, which he visited during the day, when her husband William was at work. The love between Caroline and Lord Byron consumed them, and they even had a private, mock wedding ceremony, exchanging rings and vows.

Lamb knew of their affair, and while Byron openly admired the rising political power that would one day be prime minister, the admiration was not returned. Lamb enjoyed poking fun at Byron in front of his wife, though he did nothing to stop the affair. Caroline grew increasingly obsessed with Byron, and her hysterical, high-tension personality began to grate upon the young lord. Byron ended their relationship, and sealed the deal by taking as a lover one of Caroline's friends, a much older woman. At a ball, after confronting Byron, Caroline attempted to publicly slash her wrists. Byron fled to Europe, and Caroline set to write the tale of their love. She published her novel *Glenarvon*, telling the tale of her marriage to William, and her love for Byron, the real story hidden behind a veneer of fiction. The book was published, and Lamb at last gave up on his wife, leaving her. They separated, but renewed their relationship somewhat. When Byron died, Caroline fell into a deeply destructive pit of drunken despair, and Lamb at last left her again, this time permanently, and Caroline Lamb died two years later, before her husband became prime minister, and before he was elevated to be Lord Melbourne. Thus, she is known as Lady Lamb, and not as Lady Melbourne.

William Lamb was later to become romantically involved with Caroline Norton, who was involved in one of the most infamous sexual scandals in English politics. Caroline Norton married George Norton, a Tory member of Parliament in 1827. Unfortunately for this fiery, energetic, and clever woman, her husband turned out to be a morose, dull, and sometimes violent man. Caroline began writing, as an escape from her marriage, and gained some acclaim. When her husband lost his position in Parliament, Caroline feared the consequences for her, and her marriage, of having this man around more often, and unoccupied at that. She wrote to Lord Melbourne, who was a friend of a friend, so to speak, asking if he might have a position for her husband. Melbourne visited Caroline, and the events within her drawing room during that visit have never been revealed, but have led to much speculation.

Shortly after this visit, her husband was employed, and Lord Melbourne became a frequent and regular visitor to Caroline, over the next five years, with the full awareness and consent of her now-employed husband. Norton gained political contacts through his wife's relationship with Melbourne, and encouraged it to continue. While Melbourne frequently denied their relationship was sexual, that he was her devoted fan, even "slave," was undeniable. In 1835, Norton's needs had apparently been met, and he sued for divorce, blaming Lord Melbourne for the collapse of his marriage. By this time, Lord Melbourne was prime minister, and the suit now had tremendous political implications, upon his career, and the politics of the nation. Several family servants testified to her infidelity, but the case was not proved, and Norton's allegations unsubstantiated. Melbourne was vindicated, and Norton crushed. Due to British law at the time, the Norton's could only separate, and sadly, Caroline ended up engaged in a protracted battle for custody of her children. Five years later, though her relationship with Lord Melbourne continued, she became lovers with Sidney Herbert, an aristocrat who served in the British admiralty. That relationship continued for some time, though it was damaged by other political scandals where Caroline was accused of passing political secrets to the press. When Caroline was sixty-seven, George Norton finally died, and Caroline was free. She married Sir William Stirling-Maxwell, a longtime friend and lover. Tragically, they had only a few months together, and Caroline died in 1877 at the age of sixty-nine. Caroline's story of loves, scandals, and tragedies was told in a fictionalized version by George Meredith, in *Diana of the Crossways*.

Marguerite Power Farmer Gardiner, countess of Blessington, was born in Ireland in 1789. Born in a modest family, she was married at age fifteen to a military captain, whose drunkenness and spendthrift habits led to his death in prison in 1817. In 1818, Marguerite, who had left her first husband well before his decline and death, married Charles Gardiner, the first Earl of Blessington. Gardiner had been married before, and already had four children, two by his first wife, and two illegitimate. Gardiner's first wife died somewhere around 1813. Charles and Marguerite toured Europe in 1822, and lived for a time in Genoa, Italy, where Marguerite befriended Lord Byron, and later wrote *Conversations with Lord Byron*. It was on this journey that Marguerite and Charles met a French count, Alfred Guillaume Gabriel, Count D'Orsay. The count was a friend of Byron's, and his relationship with Marguerite was quick to develop into intimacy. When Charles and Marguerite left Genoa, Charles invited the count to accompany them, and to continue his relationship with his wife. Four years later, after the trio had lived for some time in Naples, the count married Harriet Gardiner, Charles's fifteen-year-old daughter from his first wife. This marriage seems to have been an unhappy one, one that seemed intended to offer the count some financial security, and a legitimate reason for his presence in the household. The two couples moved to Paris in 1829, but Charles died suddenly, shortly after this move. The marriage of the count and Harriet ended soon after Charles's death. Less than a year later, Marguerite and the newly divorced count returned to England and lived together, the rest of their lives, though they never married. In 1849, Marguerite died of cardiac problems in Paris, where she and Count D'Orsay had fled creditors who sought to recoup money from the count. Stories of her death held that an autopsy revealed that her heart was "three times normal size," perhaps a metaphor for her capacity for love.

After Byron fled to Europe, he had several lovers. But his last lover, and the last lover who was married to another man, was Teresa Guiccioli. Teresa was born to an Italian count, and forced to marry a wealthy fifty-seven-year-old count when she was eighteen. Her husband had been married twice before, and both wives died under somewhat mysterious circumstances that led to rumors of poisonings by the count. Teresa first met Byron only three days after her wedding, but it was not until one year later, dissatisfied and disillusioned with her marriage, that Teresa began a relationship with the dashing young lord. Count Guiccioli was aware of his young wife's infatuation with Byron, and even seems to have been a confidante to Teresa, who shared with her husband the circumstances of her first romantic attractions to Byron. Guiccioli did attempt to separate his wife from Byron, taking her out of Venice, where she had met the young lord. Their relationship continued though, in heated and passionate letters. When Teresa fell ill, she begged Byron to attend her in Ravena, where she and the count lived. Though surprised at her boldness, Byron did attend Teresa there, joining her in bed, and moving into the count's palace.

Once recovered, Teresa and Byron left the palace for a return to Venice, with the count's blessings and support. The count's support was not long-lived, however, and when Byron declined to loan the count a large sum of money, or assist the count in obtaining a government position, the count confronted the couple and demanded Teresa return to their home. Teresa chose Byron over the aged husband she had never loved. The pope, asked to intervene, granted the marriage a legal separation, and Teresa then spent the next five years inseparable from Lord Byron. Byron famously inscribed a copy of Madame de Stael's *Corinne* to Teresa, describing his relationship with the book's author. When Byron went to Greece, to assist in their fight for independence, Teresa stayed behind with her father. Byron died in Greece, and Teresa appears to have mourned him for the remainder of her life. She had a few brief, unsatisfactory affairs, and married a French nobleman when she was forty-seven years old, free to marry after the count had died. Her French husband, the Marquis de Boissy, celebrated his wife's torrid relationship with Byron, introducing her as the former mistress of Lord Byron, and kept a painting of Byron in his drawing room. After his death, Teresa announced that her husband and lover were now united in the afterlife, as friends.

Throughout history, many wives and women have rejected the stricture of monogamy, or the limitation of one man to share their bed. The stories of these wives vary, with some experiencing the social punishments traditionally levied upon unfaithful women, but many have been far more successful than one might expect, given the history of severe social punishment of sexually powerful and unfaithful women. Though there is evidence that these sexual practices were not limited to the upper class, the best-documented cases are among the intelligentsia, and the literati. These women may have held some degree of insulation from social rules by virtue of their class, or by the different rules applied to artists and the creative. It may be due merely to the fact that these individuals' lives are better documented, by virtue of their artistic contributions and connections.

LES AND CINDY

*"I love you like the sun." That's what we say to each other, that
our love is like the sun.*

Les and his wife Cindy live in Utah, though they are both originally from California. I first corresponded with the couple after Cindy had kicked Les out of their house, sending him back to California. They were both forty-three years old, and had been married for around five years, living a hotwife lifestyle for almost two years. I was never able to speak with them together, and got from them their separate perspectives on their lifestyle.

Les was raised as an atheist but somewhere along the line became what he called "a Bible thumper." When he began to tell people about the sexual explorations he and his wife pursued, he found that it helped him to be closer to many of them. They now saw that he was no longer judging them but instead had "joined in the fun of being alive." Les identifies himself as bisexual, but says that this side of him has been "long-buried," though he and his wife are waiting for the right man to come along, with whom Les can "reactivate" his sexuality with men.

The couple had been fighting for some weeks, when Cindy finally kicked Les out, and told him to go back to California. This had happened before, and the couple always reconciled within a week or two. But, in this most recent incident, something different happened while Les was away. Les related that Cindy had used the opportunity to "spread her solo wings, or legs."

When Les got to California, he got an e-mail from Cindy, saying that she looked forward to resolving their issues. Still angry, Les shot back an unhelpful response. Cindy, who in the past would have headed to a cheesecake and a box of tissues, instead went to her trusty computer and arranged herself a date with a past sexual partner. All of a sudden, Les found that he was a cuckold. Before, the couple had always explored their sexuality together when other people were involved.

Les had encouraged Cindy to cuckold him, but found himself stunned that she had at last fulfilled his dreams. One of the things the couple had been fighting about was Cindy's decision to not pursue sexual relationships with people outside their marriage. She had decided that she was through with their sexual explorations, but changed her mind when Les was away.

Les described Cindy as always of two minds about sexuality. She loved many things, including being wanted and having orgasms and giving men pleasure. But she had trouble taking a stand for anything, and expressing that she liked sex was difficult. Cindy has struggled with being criticized her whole life, and often experiences it as crushing. One time, she had an instant message (IM) conversation with Les, just before Cindy left to go see the guy who was her second date, after the first time she cuckolded Les. In the IM, she started talking about what is true for her. Les feels that his wife's life is almost always a big ouch, because she is so nervous and afraid with people, and that makes her "act like an idiot" and then she ends up feeling like a fool.

According to Les, Cindy had wanted to take their sexual activity to another level for awhile, but vacillated, and sometimes wanted to simply forget the whole thing. As Cindy began to date other men, with Les out of town, she told her husband that she had decided to work on her feelings of "double-mindedness" and to just "be in the moment." Over the course of her dates, she found that she was better able to enjoy herself. She was, for the first time, able to admit to one of her well-endowed lovers that she was unable to fully enjoy herself, for fear he would thrust too deeply, and hurt her. After explaining herself, her lover was more sensitive and careful, and she ended up having two orgasms with him, which was a first for Cindy.

Cindy admitted that she is somewhat unclear on her real feelings about the couple's sexual activities. She feels disappointed with most of the men she has met with Les, feeling that they tend to be insensitive, and not interested in the kind of relationship she truly desires. Often, Cindy feels that she would be glad to just leave this lifestyle behind her, but she also feels that her sexual explorations have been the greatest gift that Les has ever given her.

Cindy acknowledged that the work she and Les have been doing has had positive impact upon her, and their marriage, aside from the sexuality. Cindy has lost weight, and taken on a new job. She feels more assertive, and more connected with her own desires for life, through her efforts to "live in the moment." The separation and the fights they've been having have helped Les and Cindy to communicate better, and to "own our own bullshit, and our sexuality." While Les was gone, Cindy had five sexual encounters with other men. On the night of her sixth date, Cindy sent Les a text message telling him she would be with another man in an hour. The encounter was intended as a thrill for Les, because she knew Les had had a particularly hard day. Afterward, she sent her husband another, more explicit text message, concluding with an expression of love for Les: "Like the sun, baby." Les explained that this meant "'I love you like the sun.' That's what we say to each other, that our love is like the sun."

Les will be returning home soon, and according to him, the couple has plans to send their "immoralities" into the stratosphere. Les recently told his wife to go on a date with a man that had been dying to get with her, but who had turned Cindy off with his arrogance and boastfulness. Les told her to go on a date with him, and have sex with him afterward. Les had never done this before, but explained that "As per our agreement, I own her sexually, and she will do anyone I tell her to and no one I veto. In exchange, I never touch another woman for the rest of my life, even in the event of her death."

Cindy shared a kind of free-form poem about one of her sexual experiences. She said that she wrote it so that her husband could share the experience, from her perspective, and see all of the things that it involved for her. It revealed so much complex internal dialogue that it is a fascinating window into the thoughts and feelings of a wife, as she offers her body to another man, with the full consent of her husband.

Cindy's story starts with her acknowledgment that she was speeding in the car, on her way to her lover's home, and that she had a secret fear mixed with desire, that she get caught by a "mythical moralistic power." When she got there, she found herself beset by insecurities about her dress, weight, and appearance, and wondered explicitly if she could "go through with this." Her lover was not deterred, however, and began to caress her. Throughout Cindy's internal dialogue, she struggled often with feelings of physical discomfort, which she restrained herself from stating, for fear of offending or upsetting the man she was with. She found herself surprised by her passion for this man, kissing him hungrily, though she said to herself that she doesn't like kissing men other than her husband. Cindy was self-conscious during their sexual encounter, but ultimately found herself responding freely to the man. At several points, Cindy found herself missing her husband, Les, thinking about him, glad that she had a husband like him, but missing the feeling of making love to Les, rather than this man.

But, Cindy gradually found herself overwhelmed by the sexual stimulation. Once Cindy and her lover were completely satisfied, and exhausted, Cindy dressed and returned home, to her life as mother and wife. She watched a movie with her son, amazed at herself, feeling the bodily sensations and scents that lingered after her experience with her lover.

Cindy's "double-mindedness" is apparent in her story, as she contemplates being done with hotwifing in one moment, and then in the next moment celebrating the impact it has had upon her sense of self, and her relationship with her husband. On the way over to him, she was speeding, excited about what was coming, but also somehow wondering if an external "moral" force would, or perhaps should, swoop in and stop her. She embraced this other man, at once conscious of the erotic feelings with him, and, at the same time, the absence of her husband. She attended to the feeling of this man inside her, yet worried about the contents of her bowels. Finally, she was both a "hotwife" and a mother, watching a movie with her child after losing herself sexually with another man. More than almost any other woman in this book, Cindy's story exemplifies the struggles inherent in this lifestyle, where a wife confronts at once all of the many expectations and burdens placed upon women, that they must be sexy, but not too sexy, must be monogamous, must be a good mother, must be moral, and must always "have their act together."

6

WIFE SHARING
IN LITERATURE
AND FILM

In 1928, D. H. Lawrence published what is, arguably, the most celebrated tale of wife sharing, *Lady Chatterley's Lover.* In this infamous
tale, Constance Reid, the Lady Chatterley, is unfulfilled by her husband
Clifford Chatterly, who is left paralyzed and impotent after the First
World War. With Clifford's urging, Constance enters into a torrid sexual
and romantic relationship with Mellors, the estate's gardener. The love
affair with Mellors was not her first, but the second of her marriage. A
first encounter with Michaelis, a playwright, happened without Clifford's
knowledge, though Connie's father had been encouraging Connie to take
a boyfriend, because living the life of a "half-virgin" was unhealthy.[1] As
Connie explored the fruits of a physical relationship with Michaelis, she
used her increased energy and liveliness to intellectually support her
husband Clifford in his own writing. In a conversation with Clifford's
peers, Lawrence began to explore the idea that sexual intercourse was
merely another form of communication between two people who intellectually stimulated each other. Through another peer, Hammond, the
idea that a wife's sexuality was the "property" of her husband was put
forth, in a manner that ridiculed and belittled the notion as an anti-
quated, uneducated relic of the past.

At last, Clifford and Connie began to openly explore the idea of her
having sex with another man, ostensibly that she might conceive a son
that she and Clifford could raise as their own, to carry on his legacy and

name. Clifford distinguished his feelings, about what sexual encounters would mean, compared to their marriage.

> But what do the occasional connections matter? And the occasional sexual connections specially! If people don't exaggerate them ridiculously, they pass like the mating of birds. And so they should. What does it matter? It's the life-long companionship that matters. It's the living together from day to day, not the sleeping together once or twice. You and I are married, no matter what happens to us. We have the habit of each other. And habit, to my thinking, is more vital than any occasional excitement.[2]

The couple began to explore this idea, this possibility, and Connie asked her husband if he would want to know about her sexual encounters. He declined, describing that he'd "better not know," but again encouraged her to understand and agree that "the casual sex thing is nothing, compared to the long life lived together."[3] Clifford encouraged Connie to take a lover, if that is what she needs, to live an "integrated" life, unaware that some of Connie's vibrant and energetic support of him had emerged from the passion she garnered from the lover she already had. It was, at this moment in their life, and conversation, that Mellors, the new groundskeeper, entered the scene, and the husband-wife-lover dynamic was fully engaged.

Before Connie pursued the sexual and romantic dynamic that had been initiated with Mellors, there had to be an end to her affair with Michaelis. A last encounter with him explored female sexuality, contrasting it with the limits of male sexuality. Michaelis chastises Connie for having to "bring yourself off by your own exertions."[4] Earlier, Michaelis had encouraged Connie to divorce Clifford, and marry him, and had been surprised by her continuing commitment to her husband. This, now combined with his sneering resentment of her sexual capacity, led to the abrupt and final end of Connie's secret affair with Michaelis.

Connie returned to the conversation with Clifford again, once more asking him if he would "mind" if she had a child. Faced with the reality of his wife's inquiry, Clifford was somewhat more hesitant than his previous intellectual commitment to the value of a full life, but agreed that she could have a child, so long as it did not affect their love. Threatened, he went on to suggest that perhaps one day, he might regain his own sexual ability, and have his own child, though it seems this comes forth as one of the darts thrown between the hurt feelings of a couple, as he does not seem to imply that this child would be made with Connie. Eventually, Connie becomes pregnant with Mellors's child. Rather than remain in this blend of two worlds, with her husband in one, and her lover in another, Connie began to dream of running away with Mellors, to marry and raise their child together. Enraged by this cold reality, Clifford castigates Connie, and refuses to grant her a divorce, that she could be free to actually pursue that ideal, an integrated life, that blends both physical and intellectual passion.

Lady Chatterley's Lover ends with the three members of the tragic love triangle separated from each other, each longing for a final resolution to the ambiguity of their circumstances. Connie, pregnant with Mellors's child, lives in Italy with her sister; Mellors works on a farm, writing to Connie, encouraging her to have patience. Clifford lives alone, cared for by a nurse, as he nurses his own resentment and anger at Connie. Clifford continues to withhold the only thing he retains of their marriage, power over Connie, in his refusal to grant her freedom. Faced with the reality of being a consenting cuckold, Clifford lost the emotional detachment with which he at first considered the idea. Faced with the reality of a love that stimulates her both intellectually and physically, Connie distanced herself from the sexless marriage to her husband, wanting both needs met in a single man, rather than in two.

Lady Chatterley's Lover, with its eloquent and detailed descriptions of the sexual encounters between Constance and Mellors, and its challenge to the idea of monogamous marriage, has been the center of numerous legal battles over pornography. (It is somewhat ironic that Lawrence himself held pornography in disregard, and insisted that genuine pornography should be banned. According to him, anything that led to the "vice of self-abuse" should be banned from public consumption.) In 1960, British prosecutors attempted to prohibit the publication of the book, arguing that British men did not want their wives to read the book. Three female, and nine male jurors disagreed, and the book was ultimately made available to the public. In 1981, the state of New York attempted to ban the film version, which starred Sylvia Kristel, famous for her portrayal as the erotic Emmanuelle. New York banned the film, as it celebrated adultery, but ultimately, the U.S. Supreme Court upheld the First Amendment, overturning the ban.

Lawrence's work may have been inspired by his friendship with the Lady Ottoline Violet Anne Morrell. Like so many other wives described here, Lady Ottoline was a woman drawn to the intellectuals of her day, and whom monogamy simply did not fit. She married in 1902, to a British politician, Philip Morrell, with whom she had two children. But, throughout their open marriage, this vivacious woman carried on love affairs with both men and women of the arts, including the philosopher Bertrand Russell, and served as a patroness to many of her artistic and intellectual lovers and friends, including Lawrence.

In the 1960s, female authors began to explore the role of female sexuality, and female infidelity, in novel ways, novel in that female infidelity did not result in automatic death, loss, or punishment for the wife. Female authors began to expound upon the value of the woman's exploration of her own sexual capacity. Erica Jong used her novel *Fear of Flying* to support this exploration, where a married woman embraces her sexuality, pursuing sexual encounters away from her husband. Coining the term the "zipless fuck," Jong idealized the physical pleasures of an almost anonymous, nonintimate sexual encounter, pursued by a woman, solely for the pleasures of the flesh that could be experienced.

Unlike most previous literature that handled issues of female infidelity, Jong's character was not traumatized, damaged, ruined, banished, or abandoned as a result of her infidelity. Indeed, it is almost impossible to find earlier examples of wives in literature who do not suffer and/or die in response to infidelity. In interviews, Jong later suggested that she had felt an internal need to punish her character for infidelity, and that it was a struggle for her to allow the character to survive unscathed, and whole.

Kate Chopin's book *The Awakening* represents the older style of dealing with female sexual infidelity, where the adulterous female character swims alone into the ocean to die at the end of the book, after having been awakened by her adulterous sexuality. Interestingly, this wasn't Chopin's only handling of female infidelity. Indeed, in a short story "The Storm," published in 1904, she described an adulterous sexual encounter by a wife, with an old boyfriend. The story doesn't end with death, destruction, and betrayal, and no families are destroyed. In fact, the female character has a lovely, happy, and healthy dinner with her family and husband, and the male lover renews his love for his own wife. Believe it or not, they all lived happily ever after.

In 2002, Catherine Millet, the author of the *Sexual Life of Catherine M*, published what has been called the "most explicit book about sex ever written by a woman." In it, she recounts not only her literally countless sexual encounters in orgies and random trysts, but also her gravitation towards husbands and boyfriends who allowed, and even encouraged her promiscuity. Millet is a well-known French art critic, who developed an early and driving interest in promiscuous sex and group sexuality. She describes many orgiastic experiences, including lying on a table in a French swinger's club, Chez Aime, while man after man penetrated her. Asked about jealousy, in an interview by the *Telegraph*, Millet's husband Jacques reports that their relationship began on very free terms, and continued so for around ten years, until they married, and Catherine began to gradually slow her sexual activities. He insisted that he was never particularly jealous or threatened by his wife's activities, and laughed that she in fact was more jealous than he, an irony he points out.

Millet's tales of her sexual exploits contain little real description of pleasure, and she even comments at one point, that in all the many, many such sexual encounters, she never experienced an orgasm during her sexual exploits. Millet said that she feels that many women have fantasies about the kind of sex she pursued, and that she differs, only in that she played the fantasies out. She is frank about her difficult childhood, but defends against an assumption that her promiscuity emerged from "neurosis."

> I was carried by the conviction that I rejoiced in extraordinary freedom. To [have sex] above and beyond any sense of disgust was not just a way of lowering oneself, it was to raise yourself above all prejudice. There are those who break taboos as powerful as incest. I settled for not having to choose my partners.[5]

But, while Millet pursued extravagant promiscuity, and found monogamy was not to her liking, she struggled tremendously with jealousy when she began to believe that her husband had himself been unfaithful. A second autobiographical book by Millet departed dramatically from the cold, emotionless tones that accompanied her tales of sexual exploits. Angst and emotional turmoil fills Millet's second book, as she wrestles with fears and concerns that her husband has a lover other than her. The two books form a striking juxtaposition, a stunning tale of a double standard, whereby promiscuity and nonmonogamy was necessary for Millet, but an unbearable proposition for her to allow to her spouse. The August 2008 *Independent* quoted Millet, saying:

> To all these people, I would say that having and living a free sexuality does not prevent you from falling into the awful trap of jealousy, and nor does it immunize you against the pain which accompanies it.[6]

Isaac Singer was a Jewish storyteller and folklorist, and a Nobel Prize winner in literature. In the story "The House Friend," first published in the *New Yorker* magazine, Singer describes learning from an older Jewish man about the tradition of a house friend. This was an arrangement, where a couple would have a male friend, as companion to the husband, and sometime lover to the wife. Max Stein is an older, semisuccessful painter and artist, who has been the house friend to several couples. In the story, Max describes to the author how this first came about for him, as he became the constant companion to a young couple when he was sixteen. Max tells how the other young man feels more comfortable with another male to talk to, and that the young woman is more talkative and pleasant to be with when receiving the attention of both men. Max tells Singer "There are men and women who don't know what jealousy is. They must share love, and besides, they never suspect anyone."[7] Another couple invited Max into their home, at first, to teach the young bride to paint, and then for more. "At every opportunity he spoke to me of how rich the soul of an artist is and how difficult it is for an artist to become accustomed to one person only. Such men are not just tolerant; they push their mates to betray them. What Feivl [the first young husband] did out of naivete, Morris did with deliberation. He wanted me to sleep with his wife, and he got what he bargained for."[8] When this young female artist fled the marriage, running away with another man, her husband, Morris, asked Max to stay around. Morris soon found another bride, whom he again shared with Max. Singer closes the story, after stating that all such men, who would share their wives, must be homosexuals. Max replies:

> The fact is that we are all searching. No one is happy with what he has. A day after the wedding, both sides begin to search, the husband as well as the wife. To me this is the naked truth.[9]

In the book *Small Town*, by Lawrence Block, several characters with intertwined lives learn to deal with the personal emotional aftereffects of the September 11 events in New York. A female character, Susan, has a ménage a trois with two businessmen. As their sexual encounters continue, she takes a more and more dominant role in the sexual activities, eventually experiencing a tremendous thrill of power as she induces the two very heterosexual men into oral, and then anal, sex with each other, completely at her direction. Even after she falls in love with one of the main male characters in the book, she continues this outside dominant relationship, at his suggestion. In the book, the male character is not threatened by her activities, and sees a healthy, empowering element in it, an empowerment that he apparently finds very, very attractive and appealing.

In 2008, Howard Jacobson, a British novelist, published *Act of Love*, a novel centered on a husband's fantasies of troilism. *Act of Love* followed Felix Quinn, as he first began to fantasize about his wife having sex with another man, and then as he began to pursue this fantasy, creating situations for her to cuckold him. Felix believed his desires were common, even universal, suggesting that all men imagine their women in the arms of other men, and that husbands are only truly happy when they know their wives are having sex with other men. This argument proliferates through the novel, with frequent references to various cuckold episodes in literary history.

Felix's desires to be cuckolded by Marisa are first sparked on the couple's honeymoon in the tropics, as he watches a handsome young doctor care for his wife when she falls ill, and is captivated by the image of the doctor's hands upon his wife's flesh. In this scene, Felix shares that "all equivocations were finally at an end, I was now someone who was aroused by the sight of another man's hands on the breasts of the woman he loved."

As a teen, Felix's first sexual encounter was when a man showed Felix the nude body of the man's wife, confined to bed by illness. Felix recounts the tale of a girlfriend he once had, who managed to "cheat" on him during the course of their first date. Felix is "successful" in his quest, able to arrange for his wife to meet another man, and to be seduced, but his pursuit of fantasy fulfillment ultimately ends in tragedy. Felix arranges for his wife Marisa to be seduced by Marius, a man perhaps best described as a "cad," a handsome but arrogant man whom Felix knows has already cuckolded another husband of their mutual acquaintance.

Jacobson has denied any personal history of troilism, and stated that he felt he would likely "die" at the idea of his wife in the arms of another man. But, he went on to say that he believed that most men actually do fantasize, to some degree, about their wives being unfaithful, and suggested that the jealousy and fears that arise from these thoughts can spur on a husband's sexuality and libido.

> Intense desire is living in constant fear of loss. Can you love someone properly, without fearing that you'll lose them? I doubt it. I doubt it. With love grows this real sense of danger. The world will take it from you! And one way to lose someone you love, is to death, or an accident, or any kind of mishap. And the other, is to infidelity, which is another kind of mishap.
>
> That corny thing where women are advised, by agony aunts: best thing to do is to make him jealous. Well, it works. It works! And if you ask me why it works, you're onto my territory. It quickens. Jealousy quickens. And to miss the quickening of jealousy, is to miss a big part of erotic life. I'm sure you can settle down and have a nice domestic life without jealousy. But—why would you want to?[10]

What I found most fascinating about Jacobson's book was not the premise, the story, or the content. Indeed, the tale of Felix and Marisa mirrors many of the literary, historic, and real-life tales of cuckoldry that I've heard and encountered. Instead, I am intrigued by the reaction of reviewer after reviewer to Jacobson's work, all of whom took issue with Felix's premise of the commonality of this desire. Reviewers such as Gerald Jacobs of the *Telegraph* described the book as literary, but reliant upon the "strained" and "outrageous premise" that men are aroused by their wives' sexual infidelity. "The desire to be cuckolded is neither interesting nor sexy. . . ."[11] Other reviewers likewise argue that it is a ludicrous idea, that husbands desire, and are aroused by, the thought of their wives with other men. The popularity of this practice, through history, and through literature, suggests that it is in fact these reviewers who may be the ones working from a false premise.

Kathy Cavanaugh, the senior managing editor of *Penthouse Letters* magazine, says that for several years, the most popular theme for stories involves the experience of sharing one's wife with another man, or regardless of sharing or not, watching her with another man (or men). Ms. Cavanaugh is quoted as saying: "If I get 30 letters in a day, 20 of them will be following that scenario."[12] The article further notes that *Penthouse* regularly dedicates a full annual issue to the topic of wife sharing. Many bookstores carry the compiled volume versions, published in book form. Volume 25, subtitled *She's Mine, She's Yours, She's Wild* and *Letters to Penthouse XXII: Views from the Top and Bottom* (*Letters to Penthouse*) are exclusively about husbands sharing their wives with other men. I learned some things, flipping through the various issues, while standing in a bookstore. First, these books seem to get read in the bookstore a lot. Buying one seemed more like buying a used book. One copy I found on the shelf had pages ripped out, presumably by someone who wanted a story, but didn't want to either pay for it, or face the checkout clerk.

From an unscientific review of the volumes of this collection, the number of "wife" letters has been on a steady rise across the years. I wonder, is the rise in response to increased demand from readers, or an increased number of such letters submitted to the magazine? In the first few pages of volume 22, the editors state: "One of the most popular themes of letters we receive is voyeurism—wife watching to be exact. It seems there's nothing quite like watching your significant other in the throes of passion with another man—or in some cases, men. Watching her gyrating, sweating, and getting off because of the ministrations and manipulations of another send your heart into overdrive and your mind into a whirlwind of erotic musings."[13]

In an interview, *Penthouse Letters* editor Cavanaugh asserted that the letters published are real, insofar as the magazine does not write them (or appear to pay for them), and the letters are submitted to them. Are they "real" in terms of recounting actual experiences by readers, or do they really reflect sexual fantasies, akin to the works of Nancy Friday? As multiple psychologists have suggested, the distinction may be irrelevant. Sexual fantasies still reveal something about people, both at an individual, and at a social level. Using these books as a kind of unscientific thermometer, the issue of wives having sex outside marriage with permission, consent, and arousal by the husband, is clearly on the rise, either in consciousness, or in open acknowledgment of the fantasy.

Among the husbands who celebrate their wives' sexuality with other men, letters published in *Penthouse* were frequently their first introduction to this fantasy, or their first hint that this fantasy was not theirs alone. Further, some found that the stories published in the magazine foreshadowed their own experiences with the lifestyle.

> Though my recollection of those stories is pretty hazy, I do remember that the guys usually described themselves being initially shocked and hurt that their girlfriend or wife would do such a thing, but then discovering that it really turned them on. Eventually I had that same bittersweet response when my own girlfriends started sleeping with other guys. Given that, I think the letters did a pretty good job capturing the emotions of this experience, even if the stories themselves were made up.[14]

On Hotwife Allie's list of books she's reading is the erotic novel *Cuckold*, by British author Amber Leigh. *Cuckold* is the tale of Edwin Miller, an extraordinarily clueless British man, who struggles for the first half of the book with the question of whether his wife Desdemona is sexually faithful to him. Much of the beginning of the book centers on the blind spot he has regarding the blatant signs of his wife's infidelities (a condom wrapper in the trash for goodness' sake!). We learn that Edwin's ability to meet his wife's voracious sexual appetite has always been less than either of them would wish. On the night of their wedding, during their first sexual encounter, Edwin "thought her needs were more than he would ever be able to meet. And, on top of that thought, he wondered how long it would be before she took a lover to provide the physical satisfaction her body required. As that question came into his mind, Edwin ejaculated."[15] For more than a year, Edwin encouraged his wife to "take a lover," after their abbreviated and unsatisfying sexual encounters. Once he finds his wife in the act though, performing fellatio on a gardener, her "Monday treat," Desdemona finally assumes command of their marriage, and their sexuality.

Desdemona confronts her husband with the reality of her sexual liberation and empowerment, and presents him with a deal. They can divorce, or they can remain together, with Edwin as her willing, compliant "cuckold," but either way, Desdemona will continue her quest for sexual fulfillment in the arms (and the sexual organs) of men other than her husband. Desdemona assumes the dominant role that she then asserts throughout the book, towards Edwin, and her other lovers. Desdemona's confrontation of her husband highlights the conflict within Edwin, and her awareness that he is aroused by her sexual infidelity, despite his other feelings of pain and loss.

> She reached across the table, as though she wanted to touch him as they spoke. He couldn't bring himself to suffer the contact, knowing that her hand had so recently been touching and stroking another man. Desdemona allowed the hand to linger between them, as though she was prepared to wait for him to respond.
>
> "I get satisfaction from other men," she continued. "And I've always known you were aroused by the thought of me being unfaithful. If we can combine these two complimentary attitudes, I think this will be the right way forward for us and our marriage. . . ."
>
> When he stared into her eyes and saw the naked devotion in her gaze, he asked, "How will it work?"[16]

Edwin's libido took a sharp upturn, as he is denied his wife's body, and is made witness to the hungry way she shares her body with others, reveling in sexual abandon and fulfillment of her enormous sexual capacity. As he watches his wife with man after man, including Jake, his arrogant, womanizing, and domineering boss, his sexuality explodes. Edwin goes from a man with a single brief sexual arousal once a week to a man who ejaculates without even being touched, over and over as he witnesses, hears, and envisions his wife in bed with others. With each new erotic challenge, Edwin experiences greater sexual arousal and pleasure. The novel ends with Edwin embracing his identity as a cuckold, arranging for his wife to spend a holiday in bed with Edwin's brother, one of her many lovers.

The website Literotica.com is a compendium of amateur erotica. The site is divided into categories, by topic. "Loving Wives" is one category of the reader-submitted stories, amongst many other categories of erotica. Other categories include "anal," "gay male," "group sex," "lesbian sex," and "BDSM," as well as about fifteen more different story themes. Of these reader-submitted stories and categories, the category that celebrates the sexual activities of nonmonogamous wives is the third largest, with nearly fourteen thousand separate stories. Only "Erotic Couplings-wild one-on-one consensual sex," and "incest/taboo—Keeping it in the family," have more stories.[17] Given that these stories, and this site, represents one of the most-visited reader-supported websites of erotica on the Internet, the role of the "loving wife" in erotica appears to be strongly on the rise, with no end in sight.

In the Oscar-winning film *Sideways*, a main character has a sexual encounter with a waitress, only to have it interrupted by her husband. The main character flees, while the husband and wife enjoy impassioned sex, apparently reliving the wife's sexual encounter.

Apparently, watching one's spouse with others is not a game merely for the living. In the film *Always,* with Richard Dreyfus and Holly Hunter, the ghost of Richard Dreyfus's character watches in anguish as his wife falls in love with another man. On her website about paranormal investigations, Gina Lanier describes this as "paranormal troilism," which she defines as "A ghost's or demon's sexual interest in watching one's regular sexual partner having sex with a third party, usually unbeknownst to the third party."[18]

Breaking the Waves is a critically acclaimed (and intensely depressing) art-house film by Danish filmmaker Lars von Trier. The plot follows the marriage of Bess and Jan. Bess is from a hyperconservative religious community in Scotland, and her new husband Jan is an oil rig worker, who brings Jan new ideas, and a novel sense of freedom from the rigidity of her community. Alas, Jan is severely injured, and paralyzed from the neck down, and soon begins to entreat Bess to tell him fantasies of her having sex with other men, due to his own inability. Lying in a hospital bed, he encourages his wife to pursue sex with other men, including his own doctor. Bess slowly begins to indulge her husband's fantasies, and the internal dialogue she carries on in the film shows that her compliance is intended to demonstrate to God her overwhelming love for Him and her husband. But Bess receives no pleasure from her promiscuity. In one intense scene, Bess masturbates an older male stranger on a bus, and then exits the bus to vomit explosively into the ditch. When she later recounts the tale to Jan, she leaves out the vomit. Bess slowly devolves into a psychotic state of depression, self-loathing, and delusion, donning a red vinyl miniskirt, and prostituting herself to sailors. Jan's doctor and Bess's family confront Jan about the devastating impact his fantasies, and Bess's subsequent behaviors are having upon his wife's mental and physical well-being. They at last get Jan to agree to never see Bess again, and secure his consent to hospitalize Bess. But Bess has already returned to the sailors, and again puts herself at their mercy. This time, they provide her the sadistic punishment she is seeking, in order to further demonstrate the depths of her devotion and martyrdom. She is beaten and raped, and ultimately dies in the hospital, though the sound of pealing bells at the closing of the film herald her admission to heaven.

In the French independent film *Romance*, directed by French filmmaker Catherine Breillat, a young Frenchwoman pursues her sexuality through many twists and turns, delving deep into fetish and promiscuity. Breillat is known as a film provocateur, and *Romance* was one of her more shocking films, including actual, not simulated, sexual intercourse between actors. Marie, the main character, feels unfulfilled in a relationship that has cooled sexually. As she begins to pursue sexual encounters outside her relationship, her boyfriend finds her more and more sexually appealing, though he is unaware of her infidelity. In one bizarre fantasy sequence, Marie, and several other women, lie on hospital beds, with their various husbands and boyfriends standing solicitously near them, as a husband would while his wife gave birth. But, instead of giving birth, the women are positioned in such a way that the nude lower halves of their bodies protrude through a wall. On the other side of the wall, roving, anonymous men touch, lick, and penetrate the women, while their husbands caress and support them on the other side of the wall. Like so many of these portrayals, however, this film ends badly for the female character, suggesting the dangerous consequences for women who reject social constraints on their sexuality.

Belle de Jour, the 1967 French film starring Catherine Deneuve, followed a sexually starved housewife who sought fulfillment as a prostitute. Her quest ultimately brought tragedy on herself and her husband, the couple condemned to a life of emotional pain as the film closes.

Indecent Proposal, with Demi Moore, Robert Redford, and Woody Harrelson, explored the similarly tragic effects of a couple where the husband, played by Harrelson, accepts Robert Redford's character's offer of a million dollars to spend the night with his wife. A classic scene in the movie occurs when Harrelson's character consults his attorney on establishing a contract, so that they don't get "screwed, and then screwed." The lawyer wasn't shocked by the husband's actions, but was instead more upset that his client had accepted what he regarded as a low initial offer.

Psychologists since Freud have examined the concepts, themes, and ideas contained within sexual fantasies, arguing that these data points offer insights into the personality and make-up of an individual. A former clinical supervisor once told me that I wasn't doing my job if I didn't have an idea by the third session of psychotherapy what fantasies a patient had while they masturbated. It took me years to realize that my supervisor wasn't suggesting that I ask, in every third session, what a patient thought about while touching themselves. Instead, he was suggesting that I needed to have developed a sufficient understanding of a given person, such that I could predict what things and themes that person would find erotically arousing. Many psychologists have suggested that erotic fantasies offer a "window" through which human psychology and sexuality can be analyzed. Likewise, literature, film, and art offers a window into the truths of human love and lives, even those truths that society would sooner not discuss.

LILITH AND TOMAS

*This, I think, is a perfect example of how kink and openness
can lead to mutual satisfaction on all sides of a relationship*

Lilith and Tomas met in a very small college in the West. Tomas grew
up in a small technological community, and Lilith was raised in an extremely conservative area of Utah, though she wasn't Mormon. Lilith was
a vivacious woman with lots of energy, and lots of cleavage. (It was apparently quite useful cleavage—she kept her cell phone and driver's license there, and goodness only knows what else was secreted away in the
depths of her bosom.) She and I had lunch a few times, and I had dinner
and visited with she and Tomas once. Lilith worked as a science teacher
and Thomas as a nurse.

While Lilith exuded energy, Tomas gave off an amazing feeling of gen-
tleness and peace. With long blonde hair, beard, and the slender body of
a long-distance runner, Tomas would easily disappear into the ascetic ranks
of a monastery. I had the strong feeling that if I were sick, I'd love to have
Tomas caring for me. I felt sure that his gentle touch and compassionate
spirit would carry me, and other patients, through even the worst illness.

Both Lilith and Tomas were sexually inexperienced before they met, in
college theater and dramatic arts. "The first time we ever started anything
kinky, where it was introduced into our marriage, was when Tomas 'accidentally' left out a video." Lilith used her fingers to frame the quotation
marks around the word accidentally, as Tomas laughed. "The video was
about men being spanked. I was game, and went to him asking if that was
what he wanted. It was, and that really started us down a pretty wild road."

Both Lilith and Tomas now identify as bisexual, though they said they've
struggled mightily to find bisexual men to share their bed. For Lilith, her bisexuality was a surprise for her. "It was at a party, and I'd never even really
considered being with a woman before. But, I played a game with people

at a party, where I went around with a bottle of liquor and told people 'trick or treat.' They could either have a shot, or kiss me. I ended up kissing up a lot of people, including women, and I went back to Tomas all worked up and pretty surprised."

Most of the sexuality outside their marriage however, involves other men. Lilith now identifies herself as a domme, dominating her husband, and other men, in BDSM activities. "As for the difference between a domme, a dominatrix, whatever . . . it's what a person decides to call themselves, I suppose. I've seen people who style themselves as a lot of different things . . . and perhaps being paid for it is a criterion between just being a domme and a dominatrix. It gets convoluted depending on whom you talk to."

Lilith identifies Tomas as a cuckold, and proudly held up her keychain for me, showing me the small key that unlocked his chastity belt, a device that worked like a cage, preventing him from achieving an erection, or masturbating. When I asked how that device worked, in their relationship, she described that they had only recently "put things together," to really understand how things worked best for them. "When Tomas is free to masturbate or have sex or stimulate himself, he has little to no sex drive. Literally. Once every week or two is plenty for him. I, on the other hand, have an extremely high sex drive, and I would have sex every day if I could, as long as *I can*. When he is locked up, he becomes attentive, caring, and has a lot of desire for me. However . . . without being able to actually have penetrative sex for any length of time, I lose interest. My libido takes a massive nose-dive and I just couldn't care less about sex anymore. You see the issue at stake here? We've come to realize that the times in our marriage when our sex lives were the absolute *best* is when I have an external partner, a man, with whom I can get the sex I crave, and still have desire to play and torment Tomas. This, I think, is a perfect example of how kink and openness can lead to mutual satisfaction on all sides of a relationship." Lilith laughed in a chagrined tone, that it had taken the couple fourteen years of marriage to reach this realization and understanding of their different sexual patterns.

Lilith and Tomas worked carefully to keep their sex lives private, at least in the community. Their two sons and one daughter were aware that men sometimes shared their parents' bed, and Lilith commented that one of their real struggles had been finding a man who was willing to have a relationship with their whole family, not just her. "I make it hard, compared to most folks in cuckolding, because I'm looking for a bull who can be hot in bed, but who is also sensitive, smart, can carry on a conversation, and has actually read a book."

Lilith, who was in charge of most of the sexuality in their relationship, said that their dream was to find a small town where they could live and work, but that was close enough to a large city that they could have a larger pool of sexual partners. "In a small town, it's just too hard. You go to the grocery store and see the parents of your students. And they are way down on their kids' teacher having any sort of sexuality." She paused, a bitter tone in her voice when she spoke again. "It's okay if you're cheating though. I know one female teacher, and everybody knows she's cheating on her husband. But nobody judges that or makes it a moral issue. But, if I want to have sex with another man, with my husband's permission, hell with him watching, that's just too much. That's just wrong, capital W.

"You know what really, really puts a screw in my gears? This whole 'discreet' thing. Oy, I swear! People say that alternative lifestyles are ruining marriage. No. They're not what are ruining marriage—cheating [husbands] too afraid to tell their wives they are kinky and want to be spanked. That's the kind of thing that is ruining marriages. Hell, half the uptight women I know would give their left breast to be able to take out their frustration on someone's ass, and have them like it. If they are so in need of understanding, then they need to get out of the playpen in their heads, put on their big boy panties, or big girl panties in some cases, if that's their particular kink, and suck it the hell up. Either be honest or stop!"

Lilith believed that it was an elementary observation that she made, as she and Tomas finally came to develop a coherent view of the ways in which her and her husband's sexual patterns meshed. I disagree. I believe that the pattern she described, where the couple had to work to maintain higher levels of sexual excitement in both of them, and where her own sexual desires diminished as she received little sexual stimulation, is a very sophisticated pattern that highlights many of the emotional and perhaps biological patterns that occur in a couple's sexuality, over the life of their marriage. Without such intense honesty and openness, over more than a decade of marriage, this couple could never have reached such a level of understanding. Most couples never do, regardless of the degree of "kinkiness" in their marriage.

7

FETISH AND
FANTASY

*The things of sex were those that most lent themselves to feelings
of horror and awe, of impurity and of purity. They seemed so
highly charged with magic potency that there were no things that
men more sought to avoid, yet none to which they were impelled
to give more thought.*[1]

Havelock Ellis

The concept of mental illness assumes that biological functioning of
the brain, personality traits, and the long-term aftereffects of significant personal experiences can dramatically change the lives of individuals, interfering in the overall functioning of these individuals as they
move through the different roles and aspects of their lives. Substantial
research has shown that most mental health practitioners assume the
presence of mental illness, when a client discloses an interest in nonmonogamous sexual behaviors. In wife sharing, this assumption emerges
in numerous ways. First, there is a core assumption that wife sharing represents a sexual disorder, called a paraphilia, commonly known as a
fetish. Second, there is an assumption that interest in wife sharing reflects the underlying expression of mental illness and personality disorder. In other words, there is the belief that the desire, interest, and practice of wife sharing are symptoms of mental and emotional disorder.

While there is a long history of research with sexual and mental disorders, much of this research, examined closely, suggests that these beliefs

161

about mental health rely heavily upon social biases and nonscientific judgment. This research often represents intent to find a single explanation for complex phenomena that actually have multiple causes. Further, an often ignored alternative explanation is that while mental health issues may sometimes be present in the phenomenon of wife sharing, this behavior may sometimes reflect adaptive responses and positive forms of problem solving. In other words, sometimes, behaviors which are uncommon may not be abnormal, but may actually be a part of a healing and recovery process.

Troilism was originally described in 1940s medical texts as the act of watching one's spouse in sexual relations with another, and noted that this sometimes occurred when the watcher was hidden. It's noteworthy that at the time, troilism was defined as a fetish. Troilism, sometimes also written as "triolism," is somewhat broadly used and is often misused merely to describe three people having sex together. There is some odd, but very interesting controversy over where the name emerged. Most speculate that the origin of the name troilism developed from the "trois" root, as in "ménage a trois." An interesting alternative explanation arises from a reference to the Shakespearean play *Troilus and Cressida*. In this work, a tragedy that follows the events of the Trojan War, the character Troilus falls in love with Cressida. Both are from Troy, but Cressida is traded to the Greeks, and imprisoned in their camp. Attempting to visit Cressida, Troilus sees a Greek soldier, Diomedes, with Cressida, as Cressida professes her love for the Greek soldier and hero. However, it seems far more likely, and supported by most references, that the term was merely derived from the Latin root of the word "three."

In the work *Sexual Deviance*, one of the most up-to-date and current diagnostic and clinical texts with regards to paraphilias and sexual disorders, troilism is described in three slightly different ways by three different sets of authors. Freund, Seto, and Kuban relate troilism to voyeurism, describing it in males as an "erotic preference for viewing or listening to one's partner interacting sexually with another man, having her disrobe where other men might observe her, or asking her to speak during intercourse about her sexual experiences with other men."[2] Kaplan and Krueger also relate it to voyeurism, referencing sex researcher John Money, and describe troilism as "A paraphilia wherein there is a dependence on observing one's partner on hire or loan to a third person while engaging in sexual activities, including intercourse, with that person."[3]

Troilism is distinct from group sex and threesomes, which may or may not constitute a paraphilia, and troilism is distinct from voyeurism in that the "person being observed is not a stranger."[4] Finally, Milner and Dopke suggest that troilism is "sharing of a sexual partner with another person while one looks on, after which the onlooker may or may not share the sexual partner."[5] Milner and Dopke also add a couple new wrinkles, referencing an author who suggested that troilism sometimes also included fathers who "arranges to observe 'his grown-up daughter' and her partner engage in sexual behavior" as well as suggesting that female troilism is rare, but not unknown.[6]

Kaplan and Krueger offer no real explanation as to the cause or origin of troilism, but Freund, Seto, and Kuban suggest "This paraphilia appears to be a transposition where the triolist pretends he is a male stranger, thus placing himself in a voyeuristic role, while his partner plays the role of an unknown person."[7] Milner and Dopke suggest there are several potential explanations, including an attempt to "re-enact the primal scene" (a Freudian concept, based upon the emotional and psychological trauma of encountering one's parents engaged in intercourse) or an "incestuous identification whereby the observer can have sex vicariously with his mother, sister, or daughter." Lastly, Milner and Dopke suggest that this behavior may emerge from "heterosexual identification with the man performing the sexual activity."[8]

I have many problems with these varied explanations, but my greatest concern is the variation itself. These experts are labeling troilism as a medical/psychiatric disorder, and yet no three of them can agree on what it is. The role of the woman or wife's desires in this behavior is completely ignored. She is either "hired" or "loaned," or, best case scenario, "shared." Finally, the idea that any one explanation, such as "transposition" or "identification," can explain all these diverse behaviors is poor science, and an incredible oversimplification of what is clearly a complex behavior. Likewise, the use of the psychodynamic processes of identification and the implied Oedipal and incestuous explanations offer unverifiable postulates based on theories that cannot be evaluated. These theories do not offer much real explanation or understanding, and create more problems and questions than they actually answer. The wide variation and disagreement about the definition of troilism is best characterized by the following point: The Texas State Council on Sex Offender Treatment defines troilism as the "use of dolls or mannequins during sexual acts."[9]

Labeling something as a disorder only works when there is agreement about the characteristics of the disorder.

Sexuality researchers and clinicians distinguish the sexual disorders of voyeurism and exhibitionism from mere fantasies by one partner, of watching their spouse have sex with another. These behaviors and fantasies occur within a stable relationship, as compared to the common history of social inadequacy often reported by clinically diagnosed (and sometimes convicted) voyeurs and exhibitionists. Likewise, one of the driving thrills for voyeurs is reported to be the fear of possible discovery, a factor not common to the spouse-watching fantasy, where consensual observation is a part of the fantasy. For the true fetishistic exhibitionist, the classic guy in a trench coat, there is a similar interest in exposing themselves specifically to those who have not consented, and are shocked and surprised by the act. The exhibitionistic and voyeuristic elements present in the activities of these couples, are no more clinical or disordered in nature than the voyeuristic urges that lead people to watch daytime talk shows, or the exhibitionistic urges that lead people to appear on daytime talk shows.

A friend of mine answers the phone for a local strip club. She told me that when the club hosts an amateur competition, the majority of the phone calls she receives are from husbands, inquiring for their wives. A large number of husbands and couples involved in wife sharing shared with me that they pursue such activities, with the wife stripping on stage while the husband watches. For the wives, they describe that they love the attention, and the exhibitionism. The husbands describe that they get a tremendous thrill from watching other men watch and desire their wives, knowing that they will get to take her home at the end of the night.

In 1990, Israeli psychologist Uri Wernik published one of the very few existing research studies regarding the practice or fantasy of troilism or wife sharing. Wernik performed a content analysis of letters submitted to an erotic magazine. Wernik argued that the issue of troilism presents a somewhat unique approach and problem-solving strategy that is utilized by some husbands and couples to overcome some obstacles in their marriages and lives. He suggested that husbands who pursue such sexual activities with their wife are quite different from the exhibitionists or voyeurs that they are often compared to. These husbands violate no one's rights, and achieve their goal, sexual fulfillment by watching their wife enjoy herself sexually with another man, by ensuring that everyone involved, wife, other man, and husband, all get their needs met. In Wernik's words, the husband shows a "certain style" in his strategies and methods, and is careful not to abuse or harm anyone:

> He enters a relationship of give and take: to his wife he gives variety and adventure without guilt feelings; to the other male he supplies sex without involvement and himself, an opportunity to watch and be watched.[10]

Wernik's analysis suggested that for most husbands, their sexual excitement was enhanced by watching or observing the other male's sexual pleasure with their wife, or by attending to their wife's sexual excitement and satisfaction. Most husbands described being present during their wife's sexual encounters, though significant numbers also participated at a distance, by watching their wife with other men in video or photographs, or by hearing their wife recount the encounter to the husband later. Around 40 percent of men had threesomes with their wife and another man, 28 percent "took turns with the other male," and 22 percent of the husbands performed oral sex on the other male.[11] Husbands who found their sexual excitement focused upon their wife's pleasure preferred to have threesomes with her and another man, while husbands who oriented toward the sexual pleasure of the other man preferred to either watch and masturbate or to perform oral sex on the other man, or both.

Nearly half of all husbands developed fantasies and thoughts about watching their wife with another man, well before they were able to manipulate the situation into occurring. These husbands often followed a pattern of introducing the idea as a fantasy to their wife, to "test the waters," and then worked to enact the fantasy if the wife was cooperative. One-fourth of the couples and husbands entered into troilistic activities as they fantasized together, in a mutual fashion, and another fourth pursued these encounters as part of their sexual repertoire when the husband discovered his wife's sexual infidelity, and found himself unexpectedly aroused and intrigued by the idea of his wife with another man.

Wernik found that an overwhelming majority of these couples found positive effects from the sexual activity, in increasing the couple's sexual satisfaction and excitement, and improving their relationships. Many of the husbands also found, and sought, a disinhibition of their wife, sexually, describing her as somewhat sexually disinterested, before the sexual encounters, with the sexual experience with other man or men liberating her and enabling her to act more freely in sexual matters. Some letters described the efforts couples made to manage the negative impact of the sexual behavior upon their marriage, with increased communication and negotiation around setting boundaries, limitations, and distinctions. Like swingers, these couples went to lengths to distinguish their activity as purely sexual in nature, as distinct from love, one writer stating, "I did not share her love, I share her vagina."[12]

Wernik proposed in his article that these sexual activities were the efforts by these individuals and couples to find mutually satisfactory solutions to some of the dilemmas of marriage. These dilemmas included: the loss of novelty and excitement in lovemaking due to long-term monogamy; the ever ongoing dance and shift of power and control within a marriage; addressing issues of male sexuality, including both bisexuality and the male comparison of oneself to other males, in efforts to establish one's value and status as a male sexual being; and, finally, dealing with the risk and reality of sexual infidelity and extramarital affairs. Wernik proposes that a husband's efforts to share his wife are often a means in which the husband finds ways to resolve these conflicts in a manner that does not destroy the marriage. By establishing and supporting this solution, the husband is able to take control of the situation, and gain some measure of control over his wife's sexuality, by the very act of setting it free from the bonds of marriage.

Wernik found little evidence to support a common psychodynamic theory, that such sexual behavior was an individual's unconscious efforts to act out and resolve the trauma of having witnessed one's parents having sex, as a child. This theory, described as the "primal scene," was relevant to only 4 percent of the data Wernik analyzed, leading him to suggest that this theory is unlikely to serve as an effective explanation for wife sharing, at a large scale.

I was able to correspond with Dr. Wernik, who has noted the rise in public popularity of troilism, and shared that he is aware of Internet communities celebrating this lifestyle, throughout Europe. Dr. Wernik feels that the increasing prevalence of wife sharing is fascinating, as it indicates the strength of "culture over evolution."[13] Husbands pursuing troilism in their marriages are overcoming a long history of murder to protect "family honor." I agree with much of Dr. Wernik's theory and research, but suggest that on this point, there's more to the story. I believe that in many ways, it is in fact the evolutionary history of sexual development that makes troilism and wife sharing so exciting and arousing for both husband and wife.

Herodotus told the tale of Candaules, king of Sardes, who was descended from Heracles. Candaules married, and had an immense passion for his wife, whom he believed to be the most beautiful woman in the world. Candaules had a bodyguard, Gyges, in his retinue, who also served as an advisor, and as a listening ear to Candaules's eulogization of his wife's beauty. One day, Candaules told Gyges that he should see the queen nude, to better believe her beauty. Gyges protested, afraid of the consequences of such an action, but the king was not to be dissuaded, and arranged for Gyges to hide in the king's bedchamber, while the queen disrobed for bed. As Gyges snuck out of the room, however, the queen saw him, and knew what he and her husband had done. The next morning, the queen sent for Gyges, and told him that he could either die for his actions, or kill Candaules, seize the throne, and marry her. That night, the two repeated the events of the night before, hiding Gyges in the bedchamber, though this time, he was armed with a knife, which he plunged into the king's heart while he slept. "Thus Gyges usurped the throne and married the queen."

Candaulism is, according to various references, the act of displaying photos, images, of one's nude wife to other men, or arranging for her to be viewed in the nude by other men, usually without her consent. This behavior may also reportedly sometimes escalate to encouraging these other men to have sexual intercourse with the wife (though, presumably, this occurs with the wife's consent). Richard von Krafft-Ebing first defined the term as a sexual disorder, in the late 1800s, in his text *Psychopathia Sexualis,* one of the first works to begin formally identifying some sexual practices as formal illnesses and disorders. Krafft-Ebing described, in *Psychopathia Sexualis,* men who attempted to share their wives with other men, including a thirty-five-year-old farmer, who Krafft-Ebing diagnosed with satyriasis (the male version of nymphomania), reporting that during this man's sexual frenzy, "He demanded that his wife give herself to other men or to animals in his presence."[14] Krafft-Ebing felt that in the social development of cultures, a turning point was reached when women were no longer regarded as chattel, but notes that part of this transition involves females developing "modesty," and becoming "conscious of the fact that her charms belong only to the man of her choice."[15] Krafft-Ebing noted that all cultures had not reached this stage, in contrast to his German homeland. He suggested that countries like Japan had only recently achieved recognition that virginity, chastity, and sexual fidelity were to be appreciated, and viewed as social and cultural imperatives. I can only assume that Krafft-Ebing was unaware of the German tradition of impotent men inviting other men to impregnate their wives, a custom formally endorsed and protected by Martin Luther, in the sixteenth century.

Despite the perceptions of swingers as emotionally or mentally disturbed, research does not support this. During the 1970s and 1980s, researchers administered various personality and psychological tests to groups of swingers and found that swingers tended to be people that leaned towards active, spontaneous lifestyles. Some studies with therapists have suggested that the individuals and couples they see that have been involved in swinging have personality, emotional, or sexual problems, though these studies probably reflect much more of the social perceptions of swingers, rather than true functioning of those involved in swinging. Overall, studies of both active and former swingers have not found that swingers have significant psychological or emotional disturbance. Such investigations are driven by what's called the "marginal hypothesis," and the idea that people who engage in unaccepted sexual behaviors are likely to be people who are marginalized in society, due to personal or social problems that have driven them to the "fringes."

The standard psychological and social explanation for behaviors such as wife sharing is to label them as the disturbed, unhealthy behaviors of disturbed, unhealthy individuals. Because wife sharing goes against the grain of so many basic Western assumptions, including monogamy, male dominance, and a prohibition against female promiscuity, it would be expected that both society and individuals would automatically condemn such behaviors. Through generalization, if the behaviors are wrong, then the person engaging in those behaviors must also be wrong, or pathological.

In this assumption, a psychologist such as myself would be expected to approach the hotwife phenomenon with theories grounded in

Freudian and behaviorist ideas. The core Freudian concept that would be applied involves the belief that individuals may gain some measure of control, or reduction in anxiety, by eroticizing a fear. Thus, masochistic urges, where an individual is sexually aroused in reaction to thoughts of being hurt or humiliated, may emerge as a response to a history of some trauma, rejection, or painful experience. Some have theorized that individuals with a history of invasive surgical procedures in early childhood may develop erotic feelings in response to thoughts of being hurt or restrained, as a way to manage and lessen the rush of bad feelings that may come with thoughts of those experiences.

So, applied to the various forms of wife sharing, this concept would suggest that this sexual interest might emerge in males in response to a strong, significant fear of their wife's infidelity. For instance, imagine a young boy whose life is tragically altered as his mother is caught being unfaithful. Their family may be destroyed, and this young boy's image of his mother is forever changed, as are his views of women and marriage. In a Freudian approach, the unconscious mind might transform these feelings into sexual arousal, to manage them and lessen the internal pain experienced. A behavioral explanation might also apply, imaging that in this boy's desperate quest to make those incredibly painful feelings and thoughts go away, he discovers that masturbation makes him feel much better and calms him. In either case, this young boy might grow up to be intensely aroused by imagining or experiencing his wife being sexually intimate with other men.

Indeed, I encountered one man, not interviewed, who presented a story almost identical to the hypothetical one described above. As a result of early family experiences, he grew up terrified that his future wife would cuckold him. He asserted that suddenly, without any real awareness, he experienced such thoughts that were extremely arousing to him, and that his fear had been replaced by a burning sexual desire to see and experience his wife being with other men. Jamie, whose interview is presented in interlude 7, described his earliest experience of sexual humiliation involving an incident when he found himself masturbating as a child, after having been bullied by other children. He grew into a man who fantasizes desperately about having his wife cuckold him with other men, particularly black men, as he is forced to watch and submissively service both wife and her male lover, humiliated by the deed, and their verbal taunting and degradation.

Dan Savage is the gay, irreverent, and very popular sex advice columnist who writes for Seattle's alternative newspaper, *The Stranger*. Savage suggests that the cuckoldry fetish is a "subconscious, erotic response to a sexually charged fear," and goes on in his column to explain that the cuckold fetish is the expression of a man's fear of his wife's sexual infidelity, conquered by the power of sexuality.[16] In typical psychological thought, this is the "eroticization theory."

While this theory may offer a compelling and intuitively satisfying explanation, it leaves us lacking in several important ways. First, and most significantly, I do not believe this theory adequately explains more than a few of the scenarios I encountered. Most described either lifelong thoughts of arousal to the idea, with no experience of any negative feelings around it, or they reported never really thinking about their wife being sexual with other men, until they just sort of "fell into it," and found that they loved it.

But, a core problem with this concept is that we do not see the approach of eroticization of fears being either common or prevalent, despite the fact that everyone, every human, by their very nature, experiences fears, anxieties, and negative emotions in their childhood and across their lives. If eroticization of fears was an effective strategy, we would see it far more than we do, which limits its general usefulness as an explanation. Many people have tremendous fear and anxiety over doing their taxes, but I don't think that many people are fantasizing about wild sex with their accountants in order to resolve these fears. This theory may explain a part of the phenomenon of wife sharing, and may be relevant in some cases, but serves best when it is combined with other theories and influences. The phenomenon of wife sharing is a complex, multiply determined behavior, where one individual cause or influence may or may not be relevant, and where many different causes are present in both individuals and the population.

Throughout the world of the modern cuckold and hotwife lifestyle, the black man, and particularly the penis of the African American male, plays a significant role. That role is one of objectification, as the black male is typically referred to as "BBC," or "big black cock." It is significant I think, that many of these couples describe their encounters with references to BBC, rather than even referring to "having sex" with someone. For many, the encounters with black males center specifically upon their penis. The role of the black male falls into an area of fetishism, referred to as an "eligibility fetish," wherein an individual has obsessive, sometimes compulsive sexual desires and fantasies about a group of individuals who would not normally be "eligible" as socially acceptable sexual partners.

Sex advice columnist Dan Savage responded to a white cuckold, who wrote with feelings of guilt and concern over his arousal to fantasies of large black men having sex with his wife. Jamie, in interlude 7, felt that his cuckold fantasies and fetish for serving black men was in some small way making up for the years of slavery experienced by blacks. In contrast, this *Savage Love* correspondent had fears that his fantasies of "well-endowed Black men" having sex with his white wife violated his progressive values and objectified black men. Savage's responses suggested that as long as this man treated these black men with respect both before and after they had sex with his wife, it is not a violation of one's "progressive" values to then watch that black man have sex with your wife.[17]

Savage's columns have generated tremendous reader response on the "slog" website regarding the racial issues. One of the most thoughtful and interesting responses came from Satadru, a black history teacher who suggested several explanations, including that the white husband was identifying with his wife, and vicariously experiencing his homosexual desire for sex with black men, by watching his wife enjoy sex with black men. Satadru also suggested that the "White man's burden" of being dominant over women and all nonwhites was a tiring load to carry. Sometimes, he suggested, white men fantasized about their wives (and themselves) with black men, as a way to "hang up his racial and gendered boots and *not* be so dominant." Finally, he suggested that the cuckold husband's desire to watch black men with his wife was another form of identification, where the husband desired to actually "be" the black man, whom the husband identifies as virile, powerful, and dominant.[18]

As I discussed this issue with couples, some identified an aesthetic value and beauty of a black man's body, and specifically, the contrast between the skin of the wife and her lover. Some couples and individuals with whom I corresponded described black men who were often better lovers, able to last longer during sex. Some commented that black men were more understanding that this was "just about sex," and were less likely to confuse the issues with feelings of love, or pursuit of a relationship beyond the sexual parameters. One contributor to OurHotwives.org described that for him, there was less perceived risk of losing his wife to a black man. While his wife might enjoy a sexual encounter with a black man, this husband did not fear that his wife would leave him for her black lover, and he could not envision his wife introducing her lover to their shared friends, or to their family. Thus, whether his beliefs were accurate or not, this husband was using the eligibility fetish as a way to manage fears and anxieties that emerge as a couple, and a wife, explore extramarital sex.

Research regarding penis size continuously generates varied results. As Kinsey (who was, reputedly, pretty well-endowed himself) allegedly suggested, the "average" penis size is always a half-inch shorter than that of the lead researcher. Nevertheless, research has largely confirmed that among the population of the United States, African American males do tend to have larger penises than other males. However, this might not be the blessing one might think. Researchers Gallup and Burch suggest that the larger penis in these men might have developed in response to the increased rates of sexual infidelity that have been found in black women. The longer penis of the African American male might be a weapon (ahem), in the sexual arms race to prevent or overcome cuckoldry, by delivering semen further into their mates' bodies, given the increased chance that their semen will be competing against that of other men. That longer penis might be a vehicle, which allows their semen to get a head-start on the competition.

Among the couples and celebrants of this lifestyle, the role of the black male is a complex, often challenging one. One black man remarked that he enjoyed the sexual popularity he commanded, and had no real problem with being a fetish object to these women and their husbands. But, he noted that the most difficult part for him was when the couples then acted as though they didn't just have an interracial encounter, and he was left feeling that if he saw the couples in public, he was unlikely to be acknowledged as a friend, much less a lover.[19] A biracial couple stated that for them, the "black thing" was racist, and described themselves as baffled and dumbfounded that "black skinned people allow themselves to be used in this way."[20]

The history of male slaveholders using female slaves for their sexual gratification is well documented. Less prevalent, but historically supported, are incidents of white female slaveholders, and the wives of slave-holders, using male slaves in a similar way. Such male slaves were often referred to as "bull dicks," a term that is almost certainly involved in the etymology of the term "bull," often used to describe black men in cuckolding and hotwifing. America's history with the black male, and his penis, is complex. Since the times of slavery, many of the crimes and assaults against African American males have specifically involved castration. This is not unique to interracial relations; castration and the taking of penises as war trophies is an ancient battle tradition, present throughout almost all human cultures. Since the first days of European contact with Africa, and the beginnings of the slave trade, black "potency" has been a pervasive myth, much of it centered on the penis. Some histories suggest that European explorers and slave traders sometimes even preserved and pickled the penises of some African males, shipping them to Europe as curiosities. Typically, the size of the African penis was held up as evidence of the "animalistic" and "subhuman" nature of the black race.

> I am informed that the Sexual power of negroes and slower ejaculation are the cause of the favor in which they are viewed by some white women of strong sexual passions in America, and by many prostitutes. At one time, there was a special house in New York City to which white women resorted for these buck lovers; the women came heavily veiled and would inspect the penises of the men, before making their selection.[21]

In 1954, in his analysis of the underpinnings of bias and racism, Gordon Allport referenced the preoccupation with sex and the black man's penis, suggesting that it was not the physical size of the penis, but the "psychological" size of the penis that was the fascination and preoccupation. In Calvin Hernton's work *Sex and Race in America*, Hernton describes the history of Southern white women's preoccupation with black men, suggesting that black males took on an iconic sexual persona. As women fantasized about sex with black men, they did so in reductionist terms, thinking of such men as "bulls," "bucks," or as a "walking phallus." These women, if they did pursue such fantasies, could transfer blame to the black male, and even psychologically absolve themselves of any guilt for their feelings of sexual attraction towards a black man, by identifying him, in real life, or merely in their fantasy, as the aggressor. Hernton suggests that the obsessive fear that some white men have, that black men are constantly sexually available to and seeking sex with white women, implies that deep in their hearts, these white men secretly yearn for the black men to have sex with their wives.

Ultimately, I suggest that the role of the black male in wife-sharing activities derives not from any special circumstances unique to this sexual subculture or practice, but from the complex history of sexual racism towards the black man. The complex, often troubling way in which black men are viewed, has to do with the history of racism in our culture. Many of the couples and individuals I interviewed and corresponded with struggle intensely with the role and meaning of black men in their lifestyle and sexuality, and do not take this issue lightly, fully recognizing the potential pain and racial stigma associated with it. Sex is not always "nice," and sexual fantasy and behavior reflects the complexity of humans, within the complexity of their social, historical, and physical environments. Sigmund Freud suggested that degradation was a common and sometimes necessary part of sexuality, suggesting that degradation was sometimes a means of overcoming fear that might inhibit eroticism.

I found the racist elements of the role of black men in this lifestyle troubling, but believe that, ultimately, we must look upon this in the same way we look at all the lingering effects of racism still present in our society. These are cues to us, regarding our history, and our future. The fact that men and women are struggling with these issues, trying to resolve their sexual fantasies, with their values and desire to treat other men and women kindly and respectfully, reflects the ongoing struggle of race and equality in our society, not a problem specific to sexual issues.

Being cuckolded is a form of humiliation, especially if one is required to be present or even to assist in the partner's infidelity. . . . The male masochist may enjoy the humiliation of being cuckolded.[22]

The cuckold relationship involves many elements common in sadomasochism, bondage, and discipline, and dominance/submission sexual practices. Indeed, the role of cuckold was celebrated by von Sacher-Masoch as a further means to experience sexual humiliation and subjugation. The sexual paraphilia of masochism involves an individual who sexually craves humiliation, degradation, and emotional and/or physical pain. Research with individuals pursuing BDSM indicates that they tend to be white, middle-aged males. Many people speculate that these men are successful, powerful individuals, who use the active release of control involved in submission as a means to escape their personal burdens. It is, at its core, according to a psychologist named Baumeister, an escape from self. Baumeister has researched masochism, showing that contrary to belief, sexual masochists are not acting out a sexualized script related to their underlying self-hatred, or desire to punish oneself for perceived internal or moral failings.

Baumeister has found that nearly one in ten individuals in the population has engaged in some form of masochistic sexual play, including spanking, slapping, and blindfolding, and that the majority of sexual masochists are males. Surprisingly, those interested in sexual masochism far outnumber those who are interested in sexual sadism, and thus many masochists develop an ability to "switch" between "top" and "bottom" roles, in a negotiated give and take that allows them to satisfy their own needs. He suggests that in some sexual masochists, the loss of control, the giving-up of control to another, reflects a relief, an escape, from the job of being an "active decision maker."

The cuckold relationship, as is intentionally enacted by the couples in this book, involves much clear, careful negotiation between husband and wife. The husband must lay out carefully what his desires and interests are, giving up control of the sexuality within their marriage to his wife, and accepting a submissive role. The wife, like the dominant in all BDSM relationships, is the one who is actually doing the work, and accepting the responsibility to meet her husband's needs and desires, and working to keep the activities within the boundaries set by the husband and couple around the sexual activities. Interestingly, research on power in (non-BDSM) relationships has found that in most heterosexual relationships, when the woman is more powerful, and the man more submissive, the couple has sex much less frequently.

Baumeister suggests that "reverse cuckoldry," wherein a female celebrates her male partner's infidelity, is almost unheard of, and argues that this difference may reflect core gender differences of one sort or another. Interestingly, aside from the practice of cuckoldry, couples and individuals in this lifestyle do not appear to pursue much other BDSM-related sexual behavior. While use of restraints such as chastity belts and sexual devices was often a component of cuckoldry-related behaviors and fantasies, the couples I met and corresponded with rarely expanded their behaviors into other BDSM activities. Indeed, when asked, few of them viewed their cuckoldry as particularly related to masochism, or at best, viewed it as a very specific, defined offshoot. Almost none of these couples or individuals described a history of practicing or pursuing other masochistic or BDSM behaviors. They did not start with other masochistic activities such as spanking or disciplining, and gravitate toward cuckoldry. Almost all of them reported their fantasies and behaviors began and ended with cuckoldry, the fantasy or desire almost "springing full-grown" into existence within their minds and lives.

The myth is that chastity belts were devices used by European knights to assure the sanctity of their wife's virtue while they were away on the Crusades. It's pretty unlikely that they were ever widely used in this manner, due in part to limitations of metal-working at the time of the Crusades. Chastity belts have been found, some used, even on a female corpse buried in Austria in the 1300s. But, the use of the belt to secure and restrict the sexuality of one's wife seems to have been somewhat exaggerated. I recall one delicious joke about a Crusades-era knight who reluctantly locked his wife in a chastity belt. But, fearing for his life and sympathetic to the idea of his wife being condemned to lifelong loneliness, the knight entrusted the key to his best friend. In the story, our thoughtful, caring knight husband got only a mile or two down the road before his friend rode up, horse in a sweaty lather. The friend waved to the knight, and exclaimed, "You gave me the wrong key!"

One recent incident involving this use of a chastity belt made the news in 2004, when a forty-year-old London woman's steel chastity belt triggered metal detectors in an airport in Greece. Reportedly, her husband forced her to wear the device as she left on vacation without him to the Greek islands, notorious hotspots for vacation infidelity, according to the British press. The pilot of the plane reportedly made an executive decision, allowing the woman to fly.

Some historical information suggests that chastity belt devices may have emerged to serve as a protective device from rapists, particularly during times of war. But, the belts came into their most widespread modern use when they were touted in the nineteenth century as devices to prevent masturbation by males and females. Some of the devices, particularly those used with adolescent males, were equipped with spikes that poked the penis if the boy had an erection. Currently though, chastity belts are enjoying their greatest level of commercial success, as they are now used widely as sexual toys in BDSM relationships, as described by Tomas and Lilith in interlude 6.

BDSM "tops" sometimes put their female and male submissives or slaves in chastity belts to prevent them from self-stimulating, or masturbating, or to require the submissive to "do without" sexual stimulation, focusing all of their attention upon the sexual gratification of the "top." Lupo, the husband of online hotwife Calliope, offered a consumer's review of his new chastity device, posting on the "Naughty Allie" site.[23] He evaluated the design and construction of the device, describing some of the issues that led to some significant discomfort for him. He noted that the fact that it was quieter than other similar devices was a boon, but noted that wearing the device constantly caused a big problem with hygiene and that, when wearing it, "I never feel clean." Lupo's big concern was that the device came only with a single key, which I have to agree is potentially a significant issue.

In 2008, German couple Jochen and Maria Ranstett, from the town of Weiden, were playing with leather and chains. They padlocked each other to the bed, but then somehow lost the key to the lock. Emergency rescue workers were called from Jochen's cell phone to the couple's embarrassment.[24] One cuckold couple told me a very humorous story of a temporary break-up in their marriage, and the cuckold husband's dismay at finding himself still locked in a male chastity belt, with his wife retaining the key. Luckily, they resolved their differences and the wife entrusted the husband with an emergency key.

Psychodynamic lore holds that women who voluntarily participate in group sex with multiple men are often pre-psychotic, with feelings of emptiness inside, difficulty knowing right from wrong, and unable to accurately define and maintain the boundaries between themselves and others. In bipolar disorder, unrestrained impulsive promiscuity, particularly among females, is a hallmark and diagnostic sign of manic or hypomanic episodes (episodes with fewer overall symptoms, or manic symptoms of less intensity). Infidelity during manic episodes has a tremendous impact upon relationships, as is discussed in detail at the website Bipolar Lives, where the woman who runs the site describes her own experience with bipolar disorder and infidelity, and the impact it had upon her marriage.[25] She cites statistics that suggest that extramarital affairs are more common among individuals diagnosed with bipolar disorder, and divorce rates are likewise higher. Among couples I met and corresponded with, in person and online, the mental health of their wives was often an important topic. Thoughtful online correspondents on the OurHotwives.org website suggested that men and couples who explore wife sharing must be as careful with a wife's mental health as they are with her physical health. Some acknowledged that some sexually exciting behaviors can be urges, driven by mental illness, rather than "authentic," carefully determined choices. Those choices, when not made carefully, can be devastating to a marriage, and a woman's self-esteem. One man described that he regretted *"having encouraged my first wife to have sex with other men while she was hypomanic."* He recognized that had she been healthy, she would have made different choices.[26]

However, few, if any, of the sexual behaviors of couples I've described occurred during periods of manic symptoms, or in concert with symptoms of other severe mental illness. Individuals diagnosed with personality disorder, such as borderline personality disorder, frequently have lots of wild, boundary-pushing sexual behaviors, as a result of their emotional and personality disturbances, combined with their craving for intense, adrenaline-fueled stimulation. But, as with true compulsive sexual behaviors, mental illness and personality disorder as severe as these would also be so severe as to prohibit the levels of positive life functioning found in these couples. Some research with bipolar disorder suggests a divorce rate as high as 90 percent, when one partner has been diagnosed. While some couples did disclose to me that some wives had histories of bipolar disorder, most did not. In particular, the many couples who shared with me that they began wife sharing after decades of marriage, had no histories of any severe mental illness or personality problems, and likely would not have reached that relationship longevity had such problems been present, much less would they have reached the point in their long marriages where they supported the wife's sexual involvement with men outside their marriage. Among those couples where bipolar disorder was present, the husbands were very sensitive, empathic, and understanding about the role of this issue in their wife's life, and sexuality.

One might speculate that the promiscuity among these wives, and the submissive, bisexual, self-defeating behavior of a cuckold husband, might derive from the long-term effects of childhood sexual abuse. However, given the staggering prevalence of sexual abuse, if the sexual practices described in this book, and nonfidelity by wives was caused by sexual abuse with any regularity or frequency, this lifestyle would be far, far more common than it is. Histories of significant sexual abuse were rarely present in the couples and individuals I interviewed. Janice, whose story is told in interlude 4, is an example of a case where an abuse history was present. But, for her, nonmonogamy was a positive, adaptive way for her to deal with her history of abuse and allow her to develop a stable relationship, rather than an unhealthy symptom deriving from the history of abuse.

Cause and effect is not an easy tangle to unweave, and the core assumption that nonmonogamy is unhealthy is based upon morals and social prohibitions, not research. A history of sexual abuse may contribute to the presence of emotional difficulty and sexual disorder in later life. But, the social assumption that sexual abuse plays a role in the development of psychopathology that contributes to sexual nonmonogamy remains an untested assumption. Nonmonogamous relationships may be, as with Janice, adaptive adjustments that help people to function in a healthy manner, rather than the reverse.

It is the effects and influence of social prohibitions, moral judgments, and fear of female sexuality that drives the need to approach the hotwife phenomenon from the core assumption that it is innately pathological or unhealthy, or rooted in negative feelings or experiences. My sample was neither extensive nor scientific, but a majority of the individuals interviewed and encountered in my investigation did not show or report such signs of negative feelings, or core personality or emotional problems. More thorough investigation could show me wrong, and demonstrate higher levels of maladjustment, but I believe the bulk of the origins and motivations behind wife sharing lie elsewhere.

In Sweden, the National Board of Health and Welfare decided in November 2008 that the behaviors associated with sadomasochism, fetishism, and transvestitism would no longer be listed as mental health disorders. Lars-Erik Holm, who heads the National Board, declared that "These diagnoses are rooted in a time when everything other than the heterosexual missionary position were seen as sexual perversions," and that "These individuals' sexual preferences have nothing to do with society."[27] Similar discussions are ongoing within the American Psychiatric Association, as they are updating the American approach to the diagnosis of mental health disorders.

The National Coalition for Sexual Freedom is advocating for revision of the American Psychiatric Association's diagnostic methodology for paraphilias, and especially for sexual sadism, sexual masochism, and transvestic fetishism. They cite research that contradicts many of the statements made within the APA's diagnostic criteria, and suggest that diagnostic criteria have been "politically—not scientifically—based. Because of this, BDSM practitioners, fetishists, and cross-dressers are subject to bias, discrimination, and social sanctions without any scientific basis."[28] Further questions as to the appropriateness of diagnosing mental disorder when dealing with the issue of transgender identification are driving the American Psychiatric Association to consider actions similar to Sweden. However, given the very different political and social climate, it remains to be seen whether such a step could be taken in the United States.

Uri Wernik suggested that troilism, and fantasies and behaviors of wife sharing, might represent a problem-solving strategy, where couples manage anxiety and fears related to possible infidelity by the wife, deal with issues of power and control within the marriage, and maintain feelings of sexual interest and excitement (working, perhaps, by means of neurochemical stimulation). I believe that Dr. Wernik's approach is a valuable one, as it forces us to consider our assumptions, and to better phrase our questions.

Rather than simply defining fantasies and behaviors of wife sharing as unhealthy, and categorizing them as sexual disorders themselves, or evidence of sexual or mental disorder, we must instead ask, what do these behaviors and fantasies do? Our definitions of sexual and mental health are changing, particularly as the fields of mental health acknowledge that many, if not most, of the sexual issues labeled as deviant and disordered had more to do with moral judgment than with research, data, or any objective evaluation. Moral judgment is a valid and important social issue, but I do not believe it effectively plays a dominant role in health care, or science. We are now learning that many people experience and practice many sexual behaviors that are not common, but are not unhealthy, and that generate no significant distress or life dysfunction. Because of the stigma and moral judgment in the medical and psychological assessments, these people simply were not seen, and remained invisible, or silent.

Even when symptoms of mental illness are present, to assume that wife-sharing behaviors are either causal, or symptomatic, also represents a potential error. The examples of this behavior among couples and individuals that have no emotional problems or mental illness must be explained before one can relate any individual problems to this lifestyle. But, like pornography, where research shows that there are tremendously and overwhelmingly far greater numbers of people who experience no negative effects from pornography use, our reaction to unfamiliar and uncommon sexual behavior triggers an automatic judgment of deviance, which generalizes to a negative judgment of a person. It is also fascinating to consider that these behaviors might, in one fashion or another, in some individuals, actually help to manage and reduce the negative impact of real mental or emotional disorder such as depression, or the lingering effects of childhood abuse. As Roy Baumeister and even the Slog poster Satadru suggest, these behaviors may serve an adaptive function within an individual and a couple, as husbands find ways to give up the burden of being in charge, and wives find ways of establishing independence and sexual freedom.

I was fascinated to read a response to one of my queries by Jason, a public affairs consultant, who described not only a positive response by a therapist, but the therapist's hypothesis as to how his cuckolding played an adaptive, positive role for his personality. This man's therapist suggested that his desires might have something to do with the man's parents' divorce, after his mother was discovered being sexually unfaithful. The therapist suggested that Jason's pursuit of these fantasies and sexual behaviors was an attempt to recreate the situation that destroyed his parent's marriage, but to give it a positive outcome, or a "happy ending." Jason's therapist took the "primal scene," and turned it on its head—Jason is trying to find a happy ending, not relive a trauma. Who doesn't love a happy ending?

JAMIE

"I am a cuckold"

Given the role of single men in the hotwife and cuckold lifestyle, I had intended to attempt to interview at least a few for inclusion in this book. Jamie wasn't the single man I envisioned, not being one of the men called bulls, who had sex with other men's wives. Instead, he was a single man, enthralled with the hotwife and cuckold lifestyle, and desperate to find a woman who could live this lifestyle with him, fulfilling his deepest desires. Jamie's first e-mail described how he had recently arranged a cuckold party, where he arranged for several wives to have sex with black men. To Jamie's surprise and disappointment, though several women and couples responded, not a single black male offered his services. Also in his first e-mail, Jamie disclosed that he had a thing for black men, a topic he expounded on in interview.

A slender white man of fifty-two, Jamie wore a Hawaiian shirt and glasses. Jamie recently retired from a long career as brewer for a beer company. He showed lots of nervous energy, and often closed his eyes as he described his sexual fantasies and urges. Whether this was due to embarrassment, or a desire to more fully enjoy the internal visualization of his fantasies was not clear. Jamie was very impressed by the hotel suite I rented for these interviews, expressing over and over again that he would love to rent such a suite, and use it for a sex party or orgy. As I described the procedures I used to protect confidentiality, such as changing names, Jamie requested that he choose the name, settling on Jamie, as it "sounds more feminine."

Jamie's marriage recently ended, after his then wife discovered he had had a sexual affair with a black man, whom Jamie met on the Internet. Jamie concedes that he is "partial" to black men, a partiality that Jamie sometimes described as a flaw, and sometimes as a fetish. "I'm obsessed with black guys. Let's turn it around. I'm the slave, they're the master. That turns me on too. And he's making love to my woman, and I wait on both of them, and am humiliated."

The Internet opened a wide world of sexual exploration for Jamie. He described how he has a problem with pornography, and the freedom of the Internet, and the availability of anonymous sexual encounters through the Internet, ultimately destroyed his marriage. Through the Internet, Jamie found that he was not the only person with these sexual desires and interests.

Jamie has been married three times. Each time, when he was first married, his "kinky" interests subsided, and went on "the back burner." But in each marriage, these desires resurfaced, and ultimately led to the termination of each marriage.

In his first marriage, at the age of nineteen, Jamie shared with his wife that he had fantasies of watching her perform oral sex on another man. His wife reacted negatively at first, but then became more accepting. The couple explored swinging for a time, until "all of a sudden, she didn't want to do it no more." Ultimately, that led to the demise of that marriage, as Jamie recalled that the couple lost their connection with each other.

Jamie's third wife did try to meet him at some level of sexual compromise. Jamie used photo-editing software to create pictures of his wife, appearing to be having sex with multiple black men. Jamie masturbated to these photos, and shared them with his wife. She told him they were very realistic, but clearly didn't find them as sexually appealing as Jamie did. About once a month, Jamie was able to entice his wife to engage in "role-playing" with him, where he would share his fantasies of her cuckolding him, and him serving her and her male lover. Jamie's wife was willing to share these fantasies with her husband, though she sometimes admitted that she was revolted by some of Jamie's desires.

But Jamie's interests in exploring the boundaries of sexuality persisted, and increased. "I started thinking of dirtier and dirtier thoughts. Like a cocaine addict, chasing that high, because, the first high, snort, it's really good, but the second one isn't, and you're chasing that first thrill. I've been through the twelve steps; I was clean and sober for twelve years. I went to AA, Alcoholics Anonymous, NA, Narcotics Anonymous, and CA, Cocaine Anonymous. I recognize that my sexual thing is a disease, an addiction."

"I'm chasing that high, because conventional sex doesn't do it for me no more, I want to watch a woman do it with another guy, while I'm sitting there in the room. Then I start thinking, Man, this is humiliating, and it's turning me on. The kicker is, the more I get humiliated sexually, the more turned on I get. She's having sex, telling him what a good lover he is, and I'm just a sissy, really putting me down."

Jamie brought out a folded piece of paper, and offered it to me. "I made up a flyer, that I was gonna give to couples, advertising me, looking for a cuckold. I brought it, but I never did pass it out, I chickened out."

I Am a Cuckold

And I am seeking a woman to share the swinger's lifestyle with me. Prefer that she plays a dominant role and be open minded to being a cuckoldress. A cuckoldress is a woman who has sex with other men, with or without her spouse's permission.

I believe it's a woman's prerogative to seek sexual pleasure in whatever way she chooses while her husband, spouse or boyfriend remains totally faithful and submissive to her. I don't believe in men to be their spouse's only option for sexual pleasure. And there is nothing that will stimulate me more than assisting you as you're taken by a real man.

Some of the duties you can expect from me:

- Help you make date arrangements for you and your lover.
- Help you pick out an outfit and dress you.
- Do anything that might make you and your lover more comfortable.
- If asked, assist you and your lover in the bedroom.

I also will be expected to do household chores such as cooking, cleaning and laundry. But I will enjoy doing them because it gives me an opportunity to serve you. Your pleasure comes first.

Since the end of his marriage, Jamie has been pursuing his sexual desires, in many different avenues. Jamie's wife read all of his e-mails, and he said she was stunned by the depths of his "perversity." As their marriage ended, because she had discovered that he was not the "the man she married," she told Jamie that he should "do what he needed to do." Some of the things Jamie feels a need to do have not worked out yet, at least not in the terms of his fantasy desires. Jamie described one recent adventure, when he went to an adult bookstore that had "gloryholes," and he performed oral sex on several men, in the store's booths. Jamie then described his recent activities to a female clerk at the store, inviting her to watch. The clerk declined, but Jamie was thrilled by her shock and surprise.

One of Jamie's most fulfilling sexual adventures was with a couple he met at a swinger's club. The wife was preparing to have sex with her husband and a black man, when Jamie commented to her that he envied her ability to arrange a tryst with a black man. The wife was intrigued, and invited Jamie to participate with them. As the wife performed oral sex with the men, she would kiss Jamie, and share their semen with him during their kisses, which Jamie called a "snowball." In the midst of the encounter, the wife turned and suddenly slapped Jamie, which he loved. The wife then wiped her husband's semen all over Jamie's face. After the encounter, Jamie tried to contact the couple, but they never responded. He suggested that it was because the encounter was "just too raw" and unrestrained.

One of Jamie's other areas of sexual exploration has been at a gay bathhouse, where he has begun exploring oral and anal sex with multiple men. Prompted by some of these male partners, he has also begun to explore cross-dressing, though he concluded that he is not interested in doing this unless he can achieve "passability" as a woman. Jamie was concerned about the risks he was taking, and the exposure to HIV. But, he reported that he wakes up each day, thinking of what he will do that day, to fill up the time. He feels his sexual desires are out of his control, and he is "willing to take that risk" with his life. He recognizes that he will need eventually to stop, but he is not ready to, even if offered an opportunity.

"Even if you said I can get you help, I know I need help but I don't want to go there yet. I know this is the disease of addiction. Anything I like, I want in excess, I chase it. The more humiliating it is, the higher it makes me feel. Sleeping on the floor, while he's sleeping with my wife or girlfriend, makes it more humiliating."

Jamie acknowledged that his sexual arousal at being sexually humiliated began at an early age, when he masturbated after being bullied by other children. He also reflected that his feelings about black men began as an adolescent, as he reacted against the bigotry of his father, having grown up in a household where "the N word was used all the time." "The root of it for me is stimulus from sexual humiliation. I didn't ask to be this way. I just am. I am not wired for a normal relationship and probably won't ever have one."

After the interview ended, Jamie again asserted that he didn't want, or wasn't ready to accept, help and stop the things that he was doing. He asked if I ever had a patient or an interviewee who was looking for a man like him, would I please tell her about him, and introduce them?

I'll preface discussion of Jamie with the statement that I don't truly believe in the concept of sexual addiction. I find it a troubling, internally confused concept that is often used to label or stigmatize socially unacceptable sexual practices in a manner that has more to do with the assertion of moral judgment than true clinical issues. Some research has shown that highly sexual individuals show no significant psychopathology or mental illness, and suggest that this label has more to do with social pressure to label illegal behaviors as mental illness. There is little clear evidence for the existence of the disorder, from a research or diagnostic standpoint, which is why the historical concepts of nymphomania and satyriasis are no longer used in current diagnostic schemes. The concepts of sexual addiction derive primarily from the views of those with social values in mind, rather than research or clinical needs. The field of sexual addiction is rife with grandiose claims, asserted with no empirical backing. As early as 1967, medical journals made claims that promiscuity was the result of cultural tension and anxiety, and an individual's inability to find worthwhile and productive things to do with their lives. Needless to say, there was no empirical evidence that showed rise in sexual promiscuity in correlation with social tensions.

While I do not support the concept of sexual addiction, Jamie does struggle with controlling his sexual urges and fantasies, and has clearly experienced significant problems and disturbance in his life due to these sexual feelings and desires. At the least, he shows clearly problematic compulsive sexual behaviors, that are endangering his life, and that he feels powerless to control. As he described, his desires and behaviors keep escalating, as he chases the "rush" of that first experience. These are patterns consistent with addictive, self-destructive behaviors. And the cuckold issue? For Jamie, it seems clear that this overwhelming desire, to find a woman to live that fantasy out, is merely another expression of this man's use of almost everyone around him, as objects to fulfill his need for sexual humiliation. A hotwife, or "cuckoldress," and especially black men, don't seem to exist for Jamie, except as two-dimensional objects, used to satisfy his internal cravings. Were he to finally sate this fantasy, it seems likely that he would lead himself, and anyone involved with him, into escalating fantasies and behaviors.

Is the hotwife or cuckold fantasy inherently unhealthy? For some described in this work, who live out these fantasies, there is a clear and deep sense of respect and regard for each other, and especially for the woman, though the outside males often seem to be seen as two-dimensional penises. Perhaps, for Jamie, it is that he lacks the ability to see himself in any healthy manner, labeling his desires, actions, and fantasies as sick, nasty, and unhealthy. Anyone who might share his desires must then also be seen through that distorting, unhealthy lens. Thus, it is likely impossible for Jamie to respect anyone else involved with him, when he cannot even respect himself.

Professionally, I wouldn't have felt comfortable without offering Jamie some support in accessing effective care. I e-mailed him, suggesting he renew his engagement in twelve-step programs such as AA, offered referrals for individual therapy to assist him in managing his feelings and desires, and recommended he consider talking to his doctor about an antidepressant. Many antidepressant medications could help him with mood, and also might suppress his libido and reduce some of his obsessive thoughts around sex.

Jamie wrote back, thanking me for the offer, but stated that he still wasn't ready to make a change in his life. Jamie had recently met a woman, interested in being a dominatrix to him, and Jamie was hoping that their relationship could at last be the one, where he could fulfill his fantasies.

8

THIS IS NO
EASY RIDE

The history of social persecution of those identified as sexual deviants is a long, tragic story. Researcher Greg Herek has shown that sexual stigma and bias is pervasive, and particularly subject to generalization, wherein if an individual engages in an uncommon or deviant sexual behavior, most people will also judge that person to be deviant and abnormal in all other aspects of their life, besides just their sexual practices. Historically, cuckolds were subjected to humiliation, and their wives to whippings, banishments, or drowning, all at the hands of their town or community. Though the methods of punishment have changed, social response to female infidelity and wife sharing remains severe.

In the 1970s, two Virginia Beach children brought family photos to school, photos that led to their parents' arrest and ultimate imprisonment. The photos showed their mother having sex with a black man, who wasn't their father. The black man was Earl Romeo Dunn, and the children's parents were Aldo and Margaret Lovisi. The Lovisi couple met Earl through a swinger's magazine, and Aldo happily photographed his wife having sex with Earl. How their daughters found the photographs is unclear, but the fact that they showed Margaret performing oral sex on both Earl and her husband was enough. Police arrested the couple, and charged them with sodomy and crimes against nature. They were convicted, and Aldo was sentenced to two years in jail, Margaret to five.

A United States federal appeals court upheld their convictions and the United States Supreme Court declined to hear their case. The trials and appeals used both the race of Earl Dunn, and unsupported allegations of exposure of Margaret's daughters to sexual activity to sway juries and judges. Although the Lovisis attempted to defend themselves as having a right to privacy regarding their sexual activity, the courts held that by taking photographs, and by having a third party present, they had waived their right to privacy. According to Appeals Court Chief Judge Haynsworth,

> If the couple performs sexual acts for the excitation or gratification of welcome onlookers, they cannot selectively claim that the state is an intruder. They possess the freedom to follow their own inclinations in privacy, but once they accept onlookers, whether they are close friends, chance acquaintances, observed "peeping Toms" or paying customers, they may not exclude the state as a constitutionally forbidden intruder.[1]

In the same year as the Court declined to review the trials of the Lovisis, the U.S. Supreme Court also denied hearing a sodomy case from Texas. Twenty-seven years later, in 2003, the Supreme Court heard another sodomy case from Texas and overturned Texas's sodomy statute.

In 1999, a Tennessee court removed custody of her child from April Divilbliss, who was living with two men. April and her male partners engaged in an open three-way, committed relationship, which they had discussed on an MTV special. According to the presiding judge, Divilbliss was "trying to have her cake and eat it too."[2] Her child was placed in the custody of the child's grandmother, despite the recommendation to return the child to the mother's custody, rendered by no less than four different court-appointed experts, all of whom suggested that the family, while different, was not unhealthy. In court transcripts, the judge characterized the relationship as deviant, and described how he couldn't "get the image of the three of them in bed out of his head." The second male eventually moved out, and the child was quietly returned to April after she declined to continue fighting the legal challenges.

In January 2005, police in Arizona raided five swingers' clubs, arresting, jailing, and fining the owners for operating establishments where public sex was conducted. Earlier controversy in Phoenix and Tucson had focused on the concerns these clubs supposedly posed with regards to prostitution, health risks, and the specific spread of sexually transmitted diseases. Operators of a commercial swingers' club in Fullerton,

California, were charged with pandering (the taking of money for the procurement of sex), and forced to register as sexual offenders.

Similar attempts to close and/or restrict swing groups and establishments have occurred in San Diego for many years. When a young girl was kidnapped and killed in San Diego in 2002, the media quickly attacked the family for the parents' involvement in swinging, alleging that their lifestyle was involved in the child's death. Even after a neighbor was convicted and sentenced to death in the crime, the parents' "deviant lifestyle" remained a frequent topic of discussion in stories and reviews of the tragedy. In Great Britain, swingers and swing clubs are prohibited or limited, with governmental and social pressure against them. In an odd irony, in both Britain and the United States, gay bathhouses have been protected by laws prohibiting discrimination against homosexuals, even though the on-premises sexual acts are similar to that which occurs in heterosexual swing clubs.

In November 2008, swingers who attended parties at a bar/hotel in Connecticut faced arrest, even after the fact. A swingers' club regularly rented-out the hotel and bar area, closing it to the public for their parties. However, police and local officials contend that because the bar holds a liquor license, it is considered a public place, even when closed. Police sent in "undercover" officers, and seized camera equipment. They declared that they had photographic evidence of the club organizer (a correctional officer at a Suffield, Connecticut, facility) and his wife engaging in obscenity and public indecency. Reports also noted that another woman was photographed performing oral sex on five men, simultaneously. Lawyers for the six defendants have stated that the arrests represent violations of their clients' civil rights and overzealous acts by "morality police."[3] In a sad irony, the town where this prosecution occurred is less than five hundred miles from the Canadian border, where swinging is now legal and constitutionally protected.

Despite these examples of social prejudice against those who pursue nonmonogamy, there is little empirical research examining these negative attitudes, as has been conducted regarding biases towards homosexuality and bisexuality. Many researchers are reluctant to undertake such research, due to the stigma that can sometimes be attached to sexual researchers, particularly in times when conservative elements in the government consistently attack sexual research as promoting immoral or unhealthy behaviors. Terry Gould describes the experience of an employee of a lifestyle organization, who had completed two master's theses on the topic of swinging, but was unable to pursue doctoral research at the University of Texas at Austin, when her research area was judged inappropriate. Research with couples and families that do not fit the mold of socially acceptable relationships might be viewed as threatening the "institution" of marriage, particularly if the research suggests that such relationships are neither pathological nor unsuccessful. Research with the nonmonogamous can be difficult, hindered by their tendency towards privacy and desire to keep their relationship arrangements confidential, as well as a desire to avoid being labeled. When I conducted very basic online research with people participating in discussions of nonmonogamous relationships, I encountered a surprising amount of healthy skepticism, with multiple people and groups wanting to confirm my credentials and intentions. I was repeatedly questioned as to whether I was approaching polyamory in an objective or biased fashion, whether I was a credible researcher, and whether I was soliciting data about sexual activities for research, or seeking descriptions of sexual activity for my own personal and sexual gratification.

What research has been conducted is extremely dated, performed primarily around swingers in the 1970s, prior to the onset of AIDS. However, even in that period, swingers were found to be perceived as deviants, whose lives reflect their deviancy. In other words, people generalize the pathology they attach to swinging, extending that pathological view towards the whole life of the swinger. Swingers are seen as drug users who are far on the liberal end of the social and political spectrum. One interesting study was done with therapists in New York, examining their attitudes towards nonmonogamous relationships, and their own experiences in relationships. Therapists perceived nonmonogamous relationships in a generally negative manner, but clearly viewed sexually open marriages as preferable to both extramarital affairs and swinging. This study was conducted in the early 1980s, and very high numbers of these therapists were in fact themselves nonmonogamous, with 40 percent reporting affairs, 14 percent had engaged in swinging, and 11 percent were in open marriages. These rates of swinging and open marriages among therapists are consistently higher than the general rates of these activities. Most studies have reported rates of some form of negotiated nonmonogamy to be around 2–4 percent, though some estimates have ranged as high as 11–15 percent of all couples. Unfortunately, most large-scale studies of sexual and marital behavior have not distinguished between infidelity and extrapartner sexual behavior that is accepted within a relationship, and there is strong evidence to suggest that couples that have such arrangements maintain them as private due to the social stigmas attached to nonmonogamous relationships. Why therapists might be more prone to nonmonogamous relationships has not been investigated, but given that this research was conducted at the end of a very liberal period in the United States, the findings may reflect social and industry characteristics that are no longer relevant. More recent research has indicated that most therapists view such relationships in very negative ways, perceiving extrapartner relationships as inherently dysfunctional.

In today's world where the lines between a shock jock radio approach and therapist are blurred by the likes of Dr. Laura and Dr. Phil, these biases remain present and significant. Dr. Phil once responded to a female caller who asked about swinging with her boyfriend by telling the woman that she would be making a whore of herself if she had sex with her boyfriend's friends.

Most of the hotwife and cuckold couples and individuals I met and corresponded with reported that they rarely disclosed their lifestyle and sexual practices to helping professionals, including doctors and counselors. One woman even expressed significant anxiety over discussing it with her gynecologist when he asked about her number of sexual partners. Given the history of judgment and assumptions regarding nonmonogamy by therapists especially, I can't say that I blame these folks for holding back this information (there is substantial research and history around similar reluctance to disclose in the bisexual and homosexual communities).

An important consideration in modern sexuality is the risk of sexually transmitted disease, especially when such diseases can carry life-altering or -ending consequences. Such concerns are an important and often discussed issue among the nonmonogamous and the communities within which they practice nonmonogamy. Some writers have argued that the strict social prohibitions against male bisexuality in swinging are an engineered prohibition to limit the risk of AIDS in swinging, and to preserve swinging as a safe activity. However, there is little evidence to support this, as it implies a directing body or individual, guiding the practices of swingers. There are bodies that loosely coordinate swinging, through managing swinger's publications and information about clubs, but there are no governing bodies that define what swinging is. While some research has shown that swingers have more concern about AIDS than the typical monogamous heterosexual couple, there is no evidence that AIDS has posed a significant risk within the swinging community. Whether the low reported occurrence of AIDS within swinging is due to the prohibition of male bisexuality within swinging or not remains to be seen. According to swinger writers, there has been a single instance in which two women reportedly acquired AIDS through repeated unprotected anal sex with two bisexual males, but there have been no published, empirical studies of the risks and incidence of sexually transmitted diseases within the context of nonmonogamous relationships in either swinging or polyamory.

Studies with polyamorous couples and individuals have reported universal concern with "safer sex," as a part of the maintaining of healthy relationships and the commitment to honesty in their relationships. Though it is important to note that most efforts towards safe sex protect users from AIDS while leaving them vulnerable to the spread of other sexually transmitted diseases. Because the "safer sex" practiced in these activities usually only involves the use of condoms during vaginal or anal sex, unprotected oral sex and other forms of nonpenetrative sexual contact leave practitioners exposed to other forms of sexually transmitted disease. Monogamy, while not suited for some, is an effective intervention and protection from sexually transmitted disease. Among other groups of nonmonogamous couples, concern for safer sex is less apparent. Hotwife and cuckold couples in particular pursue unprotected sex, and celebrate the presence and sight of another man's semen within the wife's vagina. Obviously, this does leave them open to exposure.

One correspondent to OurHotwives.org described a recent encounter he and his wife had with a clean-cut, respectful fireman, who unknowingly infected the man's wife with trichomoniasis, a common sexually transmitted disease. The husband and wife felt they had "dodged a bullet," and could have been exposed to HIV instead. The couple was unwilling to call their past behavior "foolish," acknowledging that they had made a conscious choice, but conceded that the events had led them to commit to safe sex for all future explorations.

Drug and alcohol use and abuse are typically forbidden or frowned upon within swinging, due to the risk of problems and conflict that may arise with the intoxicated during swing parties, and due to the desire to avoid "taking advantage of a drunk" in the sexual activity that occurs during swinging. Polyamorists tend to view the abuse, though not necessarily the use, of alcohol and drugs as a symptom of poor emotional or personal health on the part of an individual, and encourage that individual to pursue better health and personal choices, prior to or outside of, involvement in polyamorous relationships. Management of the risks of sexually transmitted disease that nonmonogamy carries is an issue for each individual and nonmonogamous relationship. Each relationship and the individuals involved must choose to address this concern or not, in various methods, whether they commit to the use of condoms, or choose to avoid only high-risk behaviors such as anal sex or male bisexuality. The approaches and choices vary from relationship to relationship, but it is clear that the fear of sexually transmitted disease has not rung a death knell for nonmonogamous relationships, and the risk of such disease is accepted as a manageable risk by the nonmonogamous. Like Michelle and Chris, in interlude 3, many of the people in this lifestyle moderate their alcohol use when "playing," as they feel that it detracts from the full enjoyment of the experience.

Erica Jong has said that when writing *Fear of Flying*, she struggled to resist the urge to end the book with a tragedy for the wife after her sexual adventures outside her marriage. I similarly felt a pressure to include a balancing section of this book, showing the negative consequences of this lifestyle. I encountered many healthy, happy people and couples who were pursuing various offshoots of this lifestyle. But, in the course of researching this book, I also encountered many examples where couples attempted this lifestyle, and experienced the ends of their relationships and other unfortunate outcomes that they did not anticipate when they began to explore fulfillment of their sexual fantasies. This lifestyle is no different from any other human endeavor, with two sides to each coin.

The British newspaper the *Sun* tells the story of Simon Branch, who wanted nothing as much as he wanted to see his girlfriend, Jilly, having sex with another man. Unfortunately for Simon, he got his wish. Jilly is a twenty-five-year-old blonde receptionist with striking cheekbones, a wide and warm smile, and a delectable figure. The couple had been close for three years, and lived together. Simon had made comments in the past about wanting to see Jilly with another man, which Jilly largely discounted as the fantasies many people have, but don't fulfill. But, after a late night of alcohol, Simon raised the subject again, and Jilly was willing to play along.

The two hit the Internet, invested about three hundred pounds, and within a short time, Marco Vervez, an eighteen-year-old Brazilian, was at their door. In the pictures included with the *Sun* story, Marco most resembles a young Mario Lopez, with curly black hair, olive skin, and a flashing white smile. Though nervous, Jilly soon found her nerves disappearing under the Brazilian escort's talented hands. With Simon watching in pleasure, Marco and Jilly had sex three times before the night was over. For Jilly, though, it wasn't over. The next night, she arranged for Marco to come over while Simon was out with friends. A few days later, she again paid to see Marco. And then she realized her feelings for Marco were greater than she thought. Telling Marco of her feelings, she found that this young male escort, who'd been with countless women, had developed feelings for her as well. Simon was devastated, as Jilly moved out of his home and into Marco's. In Jilly's words, as quoted in the story, "If Simon hadn't hired him for a threesome we would never have met and I wouldn't now be with the man of my dreams."[4]

In June 2008, a Swedish pastor in Stockholm had a romantic evening at home planned, involving his wife, wine, a hot tub, and a male friend. The three began to engage in what news reports called "sex games," when the Church of Sweden pastor reportedly became jealous and upset. The unnamed male friend reportedly fled the couple's home as the pastor began to physically assault his wife. According to the news reports, the pastor later admitted to assaulting his wife, but denied allegations of "kicking his wife in the genitals and slamming her head against the floor."[5] The pastor is expected to be imminently losing his job and clerical status (and his wife, I hope), though I found it refreshing that the Swedish press indicated this would result from the pastor's crimes and violence, and did not imply that the pastor's "sex games" played any role. I can only imagine that in the American press, a similar story would be likely to play up the "immoral" aspects of the sex games, in contrast to the domestic violence.

A female physician, herself a hotwife, described a recent event that ended very poorly for the "other man" involved. A couple in Dallas met a younger man in a bar, and took the man home with them after a night of flirting and text-messaged innuendo. The husband sat next to their bed, as he watched the young man sexually satisfy his wife. After the couple had both reached orgasm, the wife went to the bathroom. As she left the room, her husband pulled out a small handgun, and shot the young man in the back. The bullet lodged in the young man's back, and he is now permanently disabled. The husband was arrested, and is awaiting trial. The young man has reportedly filed a civil lawsuit against the couple, seeking financial reparations for his injury and disability.

Bill is a blue-collar worker in the Midwest, with Melody, his wife of fifteen years. Melody works as a receptionist in an accounting firm. One night, when the couple had planned to meet up with a male lover of Melody's, the lover had to cancel, and the couple instead went to a bar, with Melody's coworkers. Apparently, shifting gears was hard, and the couple ran into complications they hadn't expected.

The couple had had "simple rules," governing their sexual lifestyle, and they chose not to mix it with friends or coworkers. They also had a "veto" rule built in, allowing either of them to immediately call a halt to any activities. Nonetheless, that night at the bar, things got pretty complicated, pretty fast. A number of Melody's work friends were there, along with her boss, Tim. Melody was attracted to Tim, but given the professional relationship and the couple's' desire to preserve boundaries, they had agreed that she would not seek to have sex with him.

Nonetheless, after Melody had a few drinks, she told Bill that she wanted to make out with Tim. Bill's immediate reaction was to say no, and remind her of their rules. Melody pushed, saying that Bill should at least be happy that she had told him. Melody then asked her boss for a moment alone, and explained that she wanted to kiss him, and that "Bill was okay with it." Surprisingly, Tim politely declined the offer. Melody didn't handle this rejection well, and then followed him into the men's room. She grabbed Tim, and began to make out with him, when Bill interrupted them, taking his wife by the arm and leading her away.

Hurt, Bill told his wife that what she was doing was hurting him. According to Bill, Melody just laughed, and said "this is what you want, for me to be a hotwife, and now I'm choosing this man instead of you always picking a guy for me!" Bill took Melody home, and later that night, dealt with phone calls from their friends, all surprised at Melody's behavior. The next night, Melody blamed her actions on the alcohol, and said that she had messed up.

Later, both Melody and Bill talked to Tim. They explained that they did sometimes "play around with others," but blamed her behavior on being drunk. Tim was understanding; the three of them agreed that nothing would happen between Tim and Melody, and that this would remain a secret between them. Curiosity and concern from Melody's ccoworkers died down, and the couple set about "rebuilding" their trust. In Bill's words, the couple felt they "really dodged a bullet on this one."

A similar story was told by Jeremy, a forty-one-year-old salesman in Minnesota, who shared his own struggles with his and his wife Renee's forays into wife sharing. Despite their struggles, Jeremy continued to remain interested in this lifestyle, and wanted to find a way to make it work for him and his wife. He said that most people don't want to hear about "downers" in this lifestyle, but that he feels compelled to share his story, in order to "let people know that there are risks." He also said that there is really no one for him to talk with about these issues, because of the secrecy and the way people react.

The couple were together about four years, and married for about eighteen months, when they began "playing" with one of Jeremy's friends. They had a few experiences with him, then met another man on the Internet. A sexual encounter with him "wasn't really all that great," and the couple curtailed their behavior for about six months. Then, Renee brought up a coworker, Phillip, who had flirted with Renee, and even given her flowers once. Jeremy agreed to allow his wife to pursue Phillip, and a relationship began to develop.

Phillip came over to the couple's home a few times, hung out with both Renee and Jeremy, and so far, as Jeremy thought, things were fine. Then, he "accidentally" found out that Renee had sent Phillip a text message, and deleted it from her phone before Jeremy saw it. Jeremy confronted his wife, and found out that Renee's involvement with Phillip was at a deeper emotional level than he had been aware. He asked Renee what would happen if he told her to stop seeing Phillip, and Renee became angry, stating that she wouldn't stop being friends with him.

Things got more complicated when Jeremy went out of town on business. Renee spent almost all of the time with Phillip while her husband was away. Jeremy had arranged for Renee to call him when Phillip left their home at night. Renee did, but later admitted that she had deceived Jeremy, and that Phillip had actually stayed over all the nights that Jeremy was gone. She told Jeremy that she and Phillip hadn't had sex, and that she wouldn't have sex with Phillip if Jeremy didn't know about it. She also told Jeremy that she wouldn't sleep all night in the same bed with Phillip, because Jeremy felt that sleeping all night together in the same bed was "too intimate, and should be only with me."

The next time Jeremy went out of town, he installed a system that recorded phone calls his wife made, and also a covert surveillance system that recorded some rooms of the house. He told Renee that he was uncomfortable with her hanging out with Phillip while he was gone, but he didn't "put his foot down." "I was worried. I didn't know what would happen if I told her not to. But I also just had to know. I know it was crazy setting up the cameras and stuff, but I just had to know."

Later, Jeremy wished that he didn't know. By listening to the tapes of his wife's phone calls, he heard her tell Phillip that she loved Phillip "too much." Renee told Jeremy that Phillip was camping with friends while Jeremy was out of town, but in fact, Phillip "camped out" at Jeremy and Renee's home. He and Renee had sex repeatedly. Phillip even mowed the lawn for Renee, since Jeremy was away.

Jeremy confronted Renee, and told her that if they were going to stay together, she would have to cut off all contact with Phillip. Renee told Jeremy that she could never "hotwife" again, and blamed Jeremy for starting all this. She admitted that she had fallen in love with Phillip, but agreed to break off contact with him if the couple entered couple's counseling together. Jeremy and Renee haven't had sex with each other in months, and Jeremy said that trust was nonexistent in their marriage, and his self-esteem was "shot."

Despite these events, and the emotional impact, Jeremy continued to fantasize about sharing his wife. He felt that he could probably never again pursue the fantasy in reality, and that he would have to live "vicariously" through the online adventures of others.

Despite the prevalence of wife sharing through history and current times, there are reasons why this lifestyle is not universal. The long, long history of social prohibitions against it is not gone, nor are the social prohibitions much less relevant these days. There is a venue now, through the Internet, where these individuals and couples can explore their desires and interests, without the fear that their neighbor, pastor, or family will discover them. But, sometimes, a fantasy may just need to remain a fantasy. The emotional and relational ripples that inevitably result from nonmonogamous sexual behavior may simply be too much for many, if not most, couples and families to manage.

What does nonmonogamy mean for a relationship? To have sex with others outside a committed relationship is perceived by most in Western society to be a violation involving tremendous deception, disrespect, and dishonesty. There are numerous books published about infidelity and marriage, trying to combat the idea that an extramarital affair automatically spells the end of the marriage. Even in those Western cultures where infidelity is quietly accepted, such practices must remain covert, and when made public, are perceived as challenges to honor and respect. This belief appears to be rooted in the perception of monogamous relationships as the purest form of love, and the idea that if you're in a relationship and need someone else, then there's something wrong, either with you or the relationship. As I've counseled couples and individuals over my career, I've called this the "Disney myth," describing it as the idea that once you find Mr. or Ms. Right, you'll live happily ever after. If you ever fight, or disagree, or feel attracted to another person, then clearly this isn't "happily ever after." This belief certainly seems to support the "dooming" effect that infidelity is perceived to have upon marriages, with infidelity as the most common reported reason for divorce. Therapists and clinicians often characterize extramarital relationships as signs of discord and/or triangulation, a concept wherein an individual creates conflict between two other individuals in a way that they can use to manipulate both individuals and situations involving the three. Applying these perceptions to relationships where extramarital sexual activity is accepted as a part of the relationship may be in error. Both swingers and polyamorists have reported frustration with the perception that any problems in their relationships are always due to their nonmonogamy, rather than other unrelated relationship issues.

Most research conducted with swingers has found little difference from other relationships with regards to marital satisfaction. While many believe that the act of swinging will destroy a relationship, research has reported swingers' perceptions of swinging as generally positive and beneficial towards their relationship. Some limited and dated research with therapists has indicated that formerly swinging couples have reported problems resulting from swinging, but as there is little information regarding the numbers of couples that drop out of swinging versus those that continue participation, the ability to make generalizations from these findings may be limited. One difficulty is determining whether couples that have troubles related to swinging may have already had other, unrelated troubles.

Almost all individuals writing about nonmonogamous relationships counsel against attempting to use such relationships and activity as a way to fix existing problems in a relationship. For instance, a couple struggling with the effects or risks of infidelity or sexual problems will typically not be helped by swinging, given the complex demands nonmonogamy puts upon a relationship. Research with swingers and the polyamorous indicate that the great majority have been previously married and divorced, often due to struggles with monogamy within those relationships, and report that their current nonmonogamous relationships are far more satisfying and fulfilling than their previous relationships. The research that finds swinging and nonmonogamous couples are happy and satisfied with their relationships has been criticized as representing positive bias by the researchers, with some arguing that such couples may be engaging in self-deception or "talking themselves" into being happy with their relationship style. However, these criticisms may themselves represent bias against nonmonogamous relationships.

Some of the only empirical research about the effects of polyamory on relationships has been conducted in gay, lesbian, and bisexual relationships. While the validity of this research for heterosexual relationships may be debatable, the findings indicate that polyamory and negotiated nonmonogamy do have beneficial effects on relationships, especially when compared to relationships where infidelity has occurred. In one study with gay male couples, almost half of those couples that had agreed to be monogamous had experienced sexual infidelity in the past year.

Those couples that had negotiated agreements of nonmonogamy reported much higher levels of relationship satisfaction than couples where infidelity had occurred, even when the infidelity was still secret, with only the unfaithful partner aware of his extramarital activities.

Both swinging and polyamorous couples report a very high level of communication around their relationship needs, sexual needs, and the practice of nonmonogamy. Some polyamorous couples even have written agreements around their nonmonogamy, where they commit to use of good communication skills in and around all relationships. MSNBC writer and contributor Brian Alexander, author of *America Unzipped*, describes Kevin and Liz, a young couple whose developing, evolving rules have required much work and renegotiation. Their initial rules used state lines as a way to set boundaries, allowing sex with others when one or the other was traveling. Some sexual behaviors were okay within state lines but sexual intercourse for either of them within state lines was only allowed in the context of a threesome. Outside partners were limited to people who wouldn't "complicate" their relationship, and so coworkers and colleagues were "off-limits." But, like many other couples, no matter how often Kevin and Liz communicated with each other about their rules and limits, they found situations they didn't expect, and uncovered feelings and confusions they didn't see coming. The rules had to become a constant "work in progress."[6]

Most swinging couples report that even when they swing apart from each other, they usually discuss their sexual experiences with their spouse. Far from detracting from their sexual attraction to their spouse, they report that their "recapping" often leads to renewed sexual activity with their spouse as they become aroused sharing the details. Research with homosexual and bisexual couples that have nonmonogamous arrangements finds that the great majority do discuss some details of their extrapartner relationships, though the amount and type of information varies among individuals and couples.

Online surveys with polyamorists find that they do endorse the honesty and open discussion of nonmonogamy described by polyamorous writers, though they report varying levels of success around these discussions. Most describe their discussions with their partner as "ongoing" and "works in progress," even when they have lived polyamorous lifestyles for extended periods. Most nonmonogamous respondents seem to feel that such discussions are never quite over, and that maintaining healthy relationships requires high levels of continuing discussion. Both swingers and the polyamorous have described how their relationships were sometimes strained and challenged when nonmonogamy was introduced as a topic of discussion, but that they felt the relationship was ultimately improved as they were honest about their needs and desires. Research with both swingers and polyamorists indicates that both groups often build in time and events when they attend to the needs and health of their "primary" relationships, with time spent focusing on their emotional and sexual connection with their spouse or primary partner. Researchers at the University of Sussex found that swinging couples

> highlighted the importance of discussion and negotiation to develop a shared couple identity and shared rules and boundaries that allowed them to manage jealousy so that they could better enjoy swinging. Rather than seeking to eliminate jealousy, swingers may manage their feelings of jealousy in order to increase sexual excitement and arousal.[7]

"Compersion" is a concept defined within polyamory, as the pleasure that is found when one's partner has joy in another intimate relationship. So, the "compersive" husband or wife gains pleasure, in a deeper than vicarious sense, from seeing their partner experience the pleasures of emotional and physical love with another person.

Many swingers and polyamorists report in writing and research that their extrapartner relationships, or desire for such relationships, compelled them to communicate with their partners in a way they never had before, ultimately improving their relationship. The increased communication demands around nonmonogamy improved their ability to communicate effectively about many things in the relationship, even those unrelated to nonmonogamy. Research with monogamous couples has shown that communication, sexual satisfaction, and relationship satisfaction are linked in a complex, interactive manner that varies between couples. Levels of communication and satisfaction with sexuality and the relationship in general affect a couples' perceptions and feelings about their relationship, and research shows that the better the communication a couple has, the better their relationship in general, and the more satisfied they are with their sexual relationship. Thus, couples who have been able to successfully communicate about monogamy and relationships with people outside their relationship may be more likely to have more positive relationships in general. In contrast, researchers Daly and Wilson have suggested that many of the countless incidents of spousal homicide that occur each year in the United States are a direct result of male sexual jealousy and their fear or anger at being cuckolded by their wives. According to their research, many of these homicidal disputes start with arguments over the wife's sexual fidelity.

What about jealousy, that green-eyed monster? (Shakespeare called jealousy the "green-eyed monster" in *Othello*, and the term may have come from historical beliefs that jealousy and envy actually created a green-hued complexion.) No other issue is more consistently present across the different nonmonogamous lifestyles. These couples discuss and debate the issue of jealousy, endlessly.

Research and anecdotal reports tell us that women are more jealous of their male mates being intimate and emotionally connected to another woman, whereas men are more jealous of their female mates being physically intimate and sexual with another male. This research, much of it based upon evolutionary research by David Buss, at the University of Texas at Austin, argues that jealousy is a mechanism derived through evolution that serves different purposes in males and females. In men, sexual jealousy and possessiveness over their mate would serve to prevent cuckoldry, and limit the chances of the male using limited resources to care for another man's child. Their mate's emotional connection to another male, so long as it was not physical, would be inconsequential to the evolutionary drives of the male. In contrast, a female would care little about her male mate's physical infidelity, as any female impregnated by the male would have to raise any children that resulted, and there would be little impact upon the primary female's access to resources and supports provided by the males. However, when a male mate develops an intimate, supportive connection to another female, this would in fact challenge the availability of resources for the female mate and her children in a way that "simple" sexual infidelity would not.

Recent research by Northeastern University psychologist David DeSteno suggests that males and females may not be so different in jealousy. He found that when women have a separate cognitive task to perform, they are as instinctively jealous of sexual behavior as men. Their theory is based on research that suggests that women might be less jealous of male sexual infidelity because they believe that men can separate sex and emotion, and have a sexual relationship without developing an intimate connection. But, when women are not given a chance to think, so to speak, this belief disappears, and women respond to sexual infidelity just as negatively as men.

Males are more effective at detecting signs of infidelity on their partners and spouses, when compared to women. This emerged in a study by Paul Andrews, who found that men accurately detected about 70 percent of their female partner's infidelities, compared to the female rate of about 40 percent. But, while men were more effective at catching infidelity, they were also more paranoid about this issue than women, and erred on the side of assuming infidelity when it was not present. Researcher David Buss has suggested that the study supported the evolutionary role of jealousy as an anticuckoldry tactic in males, but other researchers suggested that the results might have to do with the simple fact that men cheated more and were thus more likely to assume their partners were engaging in the same behaviors as themselves.

Not all men are equally jealous. Men who are less symmetrical, a measure of their genetic attractiveness and value to women as mates or fathers, tend to be more jealous than their more symmetrical male counterparts. In other words, as their female mates seek out sexual opportunities with more symmetrical, more attractive, or more successful men, those men who are more at risk of being cuckolded guard their mates more jealously, to reduce those opportunities. Further, men invest more effort and resources in guarding their mate around her ovulatory period. Despite the fact that in humans, female ovulation is externally invisible, and these men are unconscious of the timing, modern males use more aggressive, controlling methods to restrict their mates' opportunities to cuckold them, when they are at the greatest risk of becoming impregnated by other men.

Could the rise of effective contraception have something to do with the ease with which modern man accepts that his wife is unlikely to be a virgin when they marry, and even the ease with which so many of the men in this book accept, or even celebrate, their wife's promiscuity? It could help, in some of the conscious, open negotiations, as couples include contraception and safe sex discussions in their extramarital sexual practices. But, at the level of the unconscious, in the gut reactions of the men, it is extremely unlikely that the presence of effective contraception for less than a century can counteract evolutionary-driven reactions honed through millennia. It is interesting to note, however, that some preliminary, unverified studies have suggested that a man releases fewer sperm during ejaculation when he is wearing a condom. Our bodies and brains may somehow know when fertilization is a possible result.

In a study conducted by Bram Buunk, it was established that men and women have different triggers for jealousy regarding their mate and a flirtatious male or female. Males respond with more jealousy when the male flirting with their mate is a dominant, powerful individual, regardless of how physically attractive the other male is. In contrast, the attractiveness of the female flirter most triggers jealousy in women, regardless of how powerful that other woman might be.

This makes powerful evolutionary sense, given that since the dawn of time, males have selected females by attractiveness, while females select males on the basis of the power, or resources, commanded by that male. Some researchers argue that this is why there are more attractive women than men, because females have been "selected" for successful reproduction on the basis of attractiveness to a degree not present in males. In other words, because attractive females have been more likely to successfully mate, reproduce, and pass on their genes, we have a higher proportion of attractive females today. Wife sharing, as these couples do it, flies completely in the face of what we know about male jealousy. These wives are engaging in sex with other males, exactly the kind of interaction that should trigger serious jealousy in the males. Further, the men in many of these couples, especially the cuckold couples, deliberately seek out very dominant males, so-called "bulls," again, in a manner that should trigger an overwhelming jealousy response by the male. Some of these couples talk about jealousy being an issue they have "worked through," and others contend that they were simply "never a very jealous person." For some, as with Earl von Sacher-Masoch, it is in fact the powerful feelings of jealousy and humiliation that are craved.

According to evolutionary theory, those individuals who were more jealous were more likely to ensure their own reproductive success, thus passing on their own genes. Jealousy then guarded the mate, protecting the female's reproductive resources from other males, and the male's protective and nurturing resources from other females. In contrast, Frans De Waal, a Dutch primatologist, argues that the social rules of shame and guilt towards promiscuity may have evolved in human society in order to level the playing field, and make the reproductive competition fairer.

Given that women are, by physiological nature, more "designed" for promiscuity, it seems somewhat more likely that the social prohibitions against promiscuity were another strategy to place barriers protecting those female reproductive resources from other males, and to preserve the parental relationship in order to support caregiving and nurturance for the children. With the modern technologies of birth control and paternity testing, these strategies are no longer critically necessary to ensure or protect reproduction.

Although we can't know whether they are feeling jealousy, when a rat or monkey mates with a female, then sees her mating with another male, he will then immediately "jump back in the saddle" and have sex with the female again, far more frequently than if the happy couple were alone, without any outside males intruding. Among humans, research has shown that when men are feeling jealous, or are concerned their female mate may have had sex with another man, they find her far more attractive, believe other men are likely to find her more attractive, and report a greater urgency to have sex with her, and, for that sex to last longer. (Recalling the studies with the smooth and ridged phalluses, and the semen analogue, those studies also showed that longer "pumping" removed more semen. Other studies have shown that women also report that when their male mate is more jealous, their sex is usually more frequent, and lasts longer.) In her work *How to Save Your Own Life,* author Erica Jong described "Kendall's first law of jealousy," that "Jealousy makes the prick go harder and the cunt wetter. It's so common you wouldn't believe it."[8]

When men watch pornography showing multiple men with a single woman, the men ejaculate harder, and their ejaculate contains more sperm than when they watch pornography with a single man and woman. If the watcher were actually present, his sperm would have to compete with the sperm of several other men, and his body and brain are responding as if the pornography is reality. Indeed, researchers Shackelford and Goetz suggest that this is the reason that Internet pornography is so dominated by images of women having sex with multiple males at the same time. Similarly, they suggest that when erotic role-playing by a couple involves the ideas of other males, it likewise triggers an increase in the male's sexual urgency for his mate, and may lead to stronger orgasms following longer, deeper thrusting.

When a male initiates urgent sex with his mate, after the female has been, or *could* have been, with another male and potentially fertilized by a male outside the relationship, the act of sexual intercourse may also serve an additional function. Additional sexual intercourse, particularly sexual intercourse that is urgent, involves deep thrusting and long-lasting penetration, and may also serve to interfere with the implantation of an embryo, if the previous sexual act resulted in conception. An interesting side note to this is that when women admit to sexual infidelity, many of them disclose that they often wait a period of time before renewing intercourse with their primary mate. Women typically share that they do so in order to conceal evidence, out of respect for their spouse, shame on their part, or simply because "it doesn't feel right." When polled on this issue, about 84 percent of women indicate they would wait at least forty-eight hours before resuming sex with their primary mate. Interestingly, the disruptive effect of sexual intercourse upon the implantation of the embryo is only effective in the first twenty-four hours. At forty-eight hours, if conception has occurred, sexual intercourse with the spouse is very unlikely to have a disruptive effect.

Jealousy is only one feeling, among many. Despite our fear of jealousy, there are many others, and jealousy may not be the most powerful. Jealousy may be overcome by other feelings, such as love, regard for the needs of the other, and altruism. Jealousy triggers activity in the amygdala, a portion of the brain that is also involved in mediating violent behavior, and initiating sexual activity. Jealousy is involved in the many acts of spousal violence. But, for some people, for unknown reasons, jealousy does not trigger a violent or angry response, or perhaps, in the sexually nonmonogamous, that response may have simply been extinguished.

In *Swingers* (published by Virgin Books, in a delightful irony), Ashley Lister explored the lives of British swingers. Lister recounts the tale of Arthur, a retired surveyor, his second wife, Betty, and their "voluntary cuckold" lifestyle. He describes interviewing Arthur in his home office, while Betty is loudly romping with a male playmate in the couple's bedroom. Arthur was in his sixties, and Betty was in her mid-forties when they began to explore the idea and reality of Betty having sex with other men. Their adventures in this lifestyle first began after Arthur developed a cardiac condition, and subsequent physical impotence. Betty had always been a highly sexual woman, and Arthur felt that he had never been able to fully satisfy his wife, due to his poor endurance, and because he reportedly had a very small penis.

When Arthur first suggested that Betty take a lover, he recounts that she "scoffed at the idea," but finally agreed when Arthur told her how much the idea aroused him, and he "showed her that the conversation had given me my first erection in more than ten weeks."[9]

With Arthur's encouragement, Betty first contacted a former lover, a move the couple agreed was a safe first "experiment." When she returned, Arthur found himself extremely aroused at the sight of her, mussed hair and rubbed-off lipstick, and the "smell of someone else's semen that was stronger than her perfume." Betty leapt full-bore into the role of cuckoldress, ridiculing her husband's small erection, and describing how thoroughly her lover had satisfied her. She denied Arthur sexual intercourse that night, but deigned to masturbate him, while she recounted in loving detail her sexual adventure. The couple's experiment was deemed a thorough success, and they continued to pursue a cuckold lifestyle. When Lister interviewed Arthur, Betty had a "little black book," filled with names and numbers of seventy-five different men, with whom she had had robust sex, for her own satisfaction, and that of her loving husband. Sometimes, rarely, Arthur was allowed to watch or listen while his wife enjoyed another man, but more commonly, she returned home and described the encounter, reliving the events of the night while she used her hand to offer her husband a physical release.

> "I can't explain why being a cuckold excites me," he admits. "It's humiliating and it should be an ordeal. My wife is sleeping with other men. She comes home from her affairs and tells me the most gory details. She ridicules me. She refuses my attentions on those occasions when I'm able to get an erection. But I wouldn't be lying if I said it's the most satisfying sex life I've ever known."[10]

Several men and couples I met and interviewed described how male impotence and medical conditions had prompted similar altruistic decisions. Alfred Kinsey's medical issues and resulting impotence may have been a motivation for his own wife-sharing activities. One couple described to me that despite the wife's insistence that she did not mind her husband's sexual performance difficulties, her husband finds "great happiness when I see her writhe in ecstasy. It's rather obvious she enjoys it." He went on to say that he is "pretty darn grumpy" at being unable to "get any," and saw no reason why he and his wife should "both be grumpy and unsatisfied."[11]

The hotwife and cuckold relationship is contradictory to the assumptions about other nonmonogamous marriages, where the belief is that the male is proposing extramarital sex by his wife, so that he can too. But, in wife sharing, the male's needs, which may be significant, in terms of the potential submissive or sadomasochistic needs of a husband who desires cuckolding, are invariably, by definition, secondary to the wife's sexual fulfillment. Linda Wolfe suggested that in her research and interviews, she found that in the various types of experimental marriages, the greatest gains from nonmonogamy went to the individual who first suggested it. In other words, she argued that when a spouse suggested opening up their marriage to include other people, the person who made the suggestion invariably had someone already in mind whom they wanted to invite into bed. In contrast, in most hotwife and cuckold relationships, while it *is* usually the husband who proposes it, the "sex objects" the husbands have in mind are for the satisfaction of their wives, not themselves.

Sluts, hedonists, and sex addicts all are terms that convey an abandon, a thoughtless, selfish drive to fulfill one's desires, regardless of the costs and consequences to self and others. In contrast to these beliefs, those involved in nonmonogamous relationships exert an extraordinary and somewhat surprising amount of energy and effort to respecting the rights and needs of others, even when they and those involved are primarily seeking nothing more than a sexual thrill. That there are ethics and principles of conduct involved in these activities takes them and those involved in them, beyond the mindless, uncontrolled orgy of self-fulfillment, and into the realm of real, reciprocal relationships. Both swingers and polyamorists report that their sexual relationships often develop into fuller relationships, involving intimacy, friendship, love, and mutual support. The risks of sexual hedonism, such as the stigma associated with sexual promiscuity and the risk of sexually transmitted diseases, have not hindered the growth or development of nonmonogamous relationships. Instead, both swingers and polyamorists have adapted to these issues, implementing different strategies to embrace, defuse, and overcome the stigma and risk of sexual nonmonogamy. Despite their different values towards love, relationships, and sex, both swingers and polyamorists appear to be acting from values that prioritize the individual need for personal growth, self-honesty, and freedom, over social restrictions governing proper, moral, legal, or acceptable behaviors around relationships.

For these couples to succeed in their chosen lifestyle, to fulfill their sexual fantasies, and maintain their relationship while doing so, requires an extraordinary level of work, commitment, and communication. Sometimes, these couples are not able to maintain what is needed to preserve both their relationship and their sexual desires. Sometimes, but not always, these couples *can* "have their cake and eat it too."

SASHA AND CHUCK

I read books and saw movies where other men enjoyed hearing about and or seeing their wives and girlfriends the same way. And then I realized that I am not the only freak out there.

In the research of Israeli psychologist Uri Wernik, elements of dominance, objectification, and dehumanization were present in the letters, descriptions, and fantasies of some wife-sharing husbands. "By making his wife do things she ordinarily would have refused and by turning her into a sex object that can be used at will" the husband "becomes dominant and in his own view, the winner in a power struggle."[1] In some of these husband's reports, themes of humiliation, group rape, and aggression were present, with husbands calling their wives "whores," or "bitch in heat," in ways that revealed significant feelings of anger and misogyny toward their wives, and perhaps women in general. Wernik found these themes in about one-fourth of the data he analyzed.

Chuck and Sasha responded to one of my advertisements, and we corresponded for a while, about their marriage and sexual activities. They sent me pictures, or at least Chuck did. Chuck initiated all our e-mail and telephone conversations. We never met, but in their pictures, they were a young, white couple in their mid-twenties. Chuck had short hair, and a stocky build. He looked like one of the young up-and-coming businessmen you see on the golf course.

Sasha was a slender, very attractive brunette, with a shy but brilliant smile. In the pictures Chuck e-mailed, they showed her posing in lingerie in front of a fireplace, and another picture showed her posing for the camera with her husband's penis in her mouth. A last photo, taken presumably by Chuck, showed the view he had looking down at his wife as he penetrated her.

They consider themselves both heterosexual, and view themselves as swingers, though they have never been to a swingers' club or participated in organized swinging activities.

When I corresponded with them, and later talked with Chuck on the phone, I learned about their relationship, but, unfortunately, only from Chuck's side. I was never able to find out what Sasha truly thought or experienced in their marriage, and can only imagine what her side of this marriage must be like. Chuck's story begins and ends with the same anger and misogyny that Wernik found in some examples of wife sharing, where the wife was treated like an object, one that was feared, and perhaps even hated.

Chuck described that when he and Sasha married, he made it clear that he would not be monogamous, but would always have his "sluts on the side," as he called them. Sasha was reportedly accepting of her husband's sexual infidelity; at least, she was at first. Chuck told Sasha that these other women would never mean anything to him, other than being "just another ho." Sasha never complained about her husband's sexual adventures with other women, and often wanted to hear about his encounters when he came home, for her own sexual stimulation.

According to Chuck, his wife is a very sexual person, who enjoyed performing oral sex and taking a submissive role in sexual encounters. He described how she enjoys being called names and being physically and verbally degraded. Chuck said that his wife especially loves the feeling of being "loaned out" to other men for sex, where she enjoyed the feeling of being "used for sex."

Chuck confessed that his own sexual thrill was other men's wives, since he was a teenager. He admitted that it was like a "drug" to him, the thrill that he got from having sex with another man's wife. He described the particular thrill he got from hanging out with a male friend, drinking or playing pool with a man who had no idea that only a few hours before, Chuck had been having sex with the man's wife. In Chuck's words, the phrase "lock up your wives and daughters" was invented to describe him.

About two years into their marriage, Sasha told her husand that she wanted to also "play." At first, Chuck refused to allow his wife the freedom to be sexual with others without his involvement.

"At first I basically said, 'no way.' I mean she is my wife, I have to keep her from doing that. But really, what could I say? I mean she let me play whenever I wanted and was cool with it. But, I still did not like the idea. Sasha liked teasing me with it, knowing how much it bothered me." There was a note in Chuck's voice here, a note that hadn't been present earlier. In contrast to his description of himself as a "sick bastard," from whom women, daughters, and other men should be protected, as he talked about his wife's desire to have other men, he sounded, for the first time, as though he was not invulnerable, and was not fully in control of his life. I imagine that Sasha probably did like teasing Chuck about this, if it was truly a "chink in his armor," and one of the only ways she could exert some control over her controlling husband.

Sasha had a crush on a younger college guy who worked out at the gym that she and Chuck went to. Chuck liked the man, but thought the idea of him having sex with Sasha was "crazy." Finally, though, Chuck gave his wife permission, so long as Chuck didn't know about it.

"So she started a fling with him. She loved it. It was very erotic for her. He would come over to our house and she and he would go into our guest room and have crazy wild sex sometimes four or five times a week. I didn't tell her, but in my mind I would go crazy whenever he would come over. I had a [ton] of emotions. Wanting to know what she was doing in the guest room and *not* wanting to know. She knew this was driving me crazy. After a few months she asked if I wanted to watch her and Mike one night. At first I just said, 'No way!' But then I got curious. I mean I wanted to see it but I didn't, at the same time. My stomach was all weird, I was turned on and sick to my gut, at the same time."

One night, Sasha got the impression that Chuck wanted to watch her with her lover but wouldn't, or couldn't, admit it. Mike came over and they went right into the guest room. Sasha left the curtains open in the guestroom, so that if Chuck were in their bedroom, he could look out the window and into the guestroom.

An hour later, Chuck found himself glued to the window, watching his wife have sex with her lover. Her lover knew that Chuck was watching, and worked hard to "put on a show," displaying the degree of sexual dominance he had over her.

Chuck's conflicted emotions continued. "I was crazy in my mind. She loved it. And you could tell by the look on his face that he loved doing this knowing I was watching. I understood and knew the 'high' he got from this because I had done it with so many other men's wives before. And my wife was loving it. You could tell he knew what she liked. He was degrading her, calling her dirty names and slapping her ass and pulling her hair.

"Again I had all these crazy emotions. I guess the biggest thing for me was feeling guilty because I enjoyed seeing what I was seeing when she was with him. I mean I thought I was crazy because I should not be enjoying seeing my wife like this. But later, I read books and saw movies where other men enjoyed hearing about and/or seeing their wives and girlfriends the same way. And then I realized that I am not the only freak out there."

Sasha's relationship with this man continued, and expanded to include the man's roommate. The two men treated Sasha as their whore, and would stop by their house late at night to use her sexually, in a way that Chuck, and his wife, found extremely exciting.

Sasha continued to see Mike and his roommate, Kyle, for about a year. It improved her sex life with Chuck, in ways the couple hadn't anticipated. Mostly they came over, one at a time, at different times. They would call her and tell her what time one of them would be there and Sasha would wait for them in the guest room.

Chuck worked early in the mornings, and often he and his wife would have sex and go to bed. He would awaken at two or three in the morning, and she would be gone. When Chuck looked out the window, into the guest room, he would see his wife with one of the other men.

On two occasions, Mike and Kyle brought other men to share Sasha. Once, they brought a male cousin to Sasha to lose his virginity, and another time they brought a male friend to her, during his bachelor party, for a "last sexual experience before getting married." Sasha found these experiences very erotic, as she was treated as a sexual plaything.

This relationship lasted about two years, until the two young men finished college and moved away. Chuck and Sasha are still looking for other men to share her with. Chuck continues to pursue other men's wives, but has found that the idea of sharing his own wife is far more arousing than he had ever imagined.

Chuck and Sasha didn't keep our scheduled meeting, and I never heard from them afterward. When I posted an advertisement on Craigslist, I usually posted a photo of myself, for a few reasons. Mostly, I learned that many people who scan Craigslist preferentially look at advertisements with a photo attached. Second, I wanted people to see that I was a real person, and so that they could recognize me when we met. Chuck and Sasha apparently thought my photo and advertisement offered the possibility of something else. As we corresponded, Chuck often told me that his wife wanted to see more photos of me, and that she was enjoying the idea of us meeting. I was always careful, in my responses, to indicate that I too looked forward to our meeting, so that I could hear more "about the way their marriage worked." I have to assume that they weren't really interested in "my mind," though, and that Chuck was really looking for a situation where I would get to know his wife in a far different way.

I saw very little misogyny in the hotwife lifestyle, despite the assumption that it would be prevalent, and that the lifestyle revolved around men treating their wives as property. As I've discussed, the role of wives, and female sexuality, as a form of property has an incredibly long and varied history throughout all corners of the globe. Sadly, there is nothing new about men treating their wives as objects, to be given away, degraded, or used for the husband's own needs. I think it is significant that Chuck and Sasha were not involved in any of the organized groups around swinging or hotwifing, where misogyny as blatant as Chuck's receives little tolerance.

Chuck, with his attitudes towards other women, and his own wife, seemed to have a great fear of women, and a need to bring them down a peg. Somewhere, for some reason, this man ended up with a deep, driving need to subjugate women to his sexual desires, and to use women to weaken and undermine other men. And for some reason, his wife ended up with the willingness to comply. Her effort to connect with her husband even more deeply led her to find a way that she could become just like one of the wives that her husband was fixated upon.

A more sophisticated issue is implicit in Chuck's willingness to allow other men to do to his wife what he does to other men and their wives. In doing so, Chuck relinquished, briefly, his "tough guy" persona, and accepted the experience of not being in charge. For a time, Chuck was able to experience being vulnerable, to experience his wife having independence from him, and to experience other men being dominant over him. And he was able to survive these experiences in a way that he probably would have previously believed he could not.

9

A WILD NEW WORLD OF WIFE SHARING

For those who wish to control others' sexuality, thinking, or family structure, the Internet is a nightmare come true.

Marty Klein, Ph.D.[1]

Like almost everything else in the world, the various types of wife sharing have embraced and changed technology, and been changed by it. In the most dramatic shift, thanks to the democratic power of the Internet, wife-sharing activities are now widely acknowledged and celebrated. Now, thanks to the literally awesome power of a Google search, an interested man or woman can perform a literature search in seconds that would previously have taken months. An individual with a momentary fantasy of sharing his wife can instantly find photographs, videos, stories, and forums that offer him the knowledge that he is not alone in this fantasy, and that there are many others out there who have made this fantasy a reality. Might these experiences feed this fantasy, and fan the flames to life around an ember that might have flickered briefly and died?

A fascinating modern derivative of candaulism is now available, thanks to the wonders of digital photography. Many Internet sites offer visitors the opportunity to post photos of their wives, and view photos of the wives of other visitors. But, mere posting of nude photos of one's wife has become almost passé. Now, men post pictures of their wife online, requesting other men do things such as reposting the pictures elsewhere online. Some request that others print out pictures of the wife and physically place them out in public, where others can see, and take pictures of the photo out in public. Others request that men take pictures of themselves masturbating and ejaculating onto their wife's photo and repost those pictures. On the bulletin board of the site Voyeurweb.com, men (and sometimes couples, apparently) sometimes ask other group members to repost photos of their wife that these other members have saved, in a way of demonstrating, perhaps, that the wife is desirable enough to be "collected" by other men.

When asked about the appeal of this practice, one man responded to me that:

> I like to see erotically dressed women, the more the better. Husbands don't post their wives' images in a vacuum; they do it for feedback. I think it's a progression toward a certain mode of thinking, a way of life that just happens to offend the hysterical moral majority. Tough shit— beautifully erotic bodies were around long before the edict to cover them up. A picture is not wife sharing, that's something else entirely. But the two ideals are similarly offensive to the masses and that sweetens the cerebral pot for us non-conformists.

He then added a quote from de Sade:

> The imagination is the spur of delights . . . all depends upon it, it is the mainspring of everything; now, is it not by the means of the imagination one knows joy? Is it not of the imagination that the sharpest pleasures arise?[2]

Thanks to the capabilities of photo-editing software, a husband does not even need his wife to pose nude. Makers of altered photos invite husbands to participate, telling them that if the husbands provide photographs of their wife's face, they will create nude photographs of her for the husband's enjoyment.[3]

As Jamie describes in interlude 7, some men take existing photos of their wives and manipulate them to appear as if the wife was engaging in sex with other men, using pornographic pictures and photo-altering software to create fantasy photographs. Some report that the altered photographs become a part of their fantasy play, which sometimes even contributes toward the possibility of turning their fantasies into reality.[4]

A maker of many of these electronic creations, which I guess could be called a form of digital art, uses the name "Photoshop Phantasees" for his work. I corresponded with him, trying to understand the motivations for his activities. He replied that:

> Guys are visually oriented (and not too good with imagination LOL) so seeing what they fantasize about makes, for some, a stronger fantasy. Plus there is the surprise of what someone else will do with their wife, in a picture, or maybe even in reality.
>
> Personally, I do it because I have a fetish of being the only guy besides her doctor and husband to see her naked body. Obviously not the requests made on bulletin boards online, but from the lurkers who never post their sweetie online. They trust me to keep photos they e-mail to me private. I also get to see the beautiful eyes and faces of many ladies who are posted blurred or cropped.[5]

Some men and women request to see their photographs not manipulated, but posted in public, for the world to see, requesting they be posted on places like state signs, in department stores, and elevators.[6] One person replied with some cautious advice, which I expect is appreciated by those of us who are parents. He suggested that, while he was open to location suggestions, he doesn't leave R- or X-rated pictures in public locations where they could be seen by children. Instead, he posts in places like liquor stores, men's restrooms in bars, and adult sex stores.[7]

Of course, for every wife out there who allows, supports, or pursues these activities, with or without her husband, there are many more who adamantly refuse. Not that this necessarily prevents it from happening, in one way or another. One posting I saw on Craigslist was from a man whose "hot soccer mom" wife would not fulfill his fantasy of her having sex with other men. So, this husband pursued "the next best thing," and invited other men to masturbate with him, while they looked at photographs of his wife, and talked about the men having sex with her.[8]

A Google search for the terms "cuckold" or "hotwife" generates a tremendous number of sites, with porn galore. One of the more clever links was to the home of self-styled "Cuckold Queen" Candy Monroe. Candy was a tattooed blonde, surprisingly pretty in a classic 1950s pin-up style, glossy hair reminiscent of Veronica Lake. Candy welcomes visitors to her site with numerous pictures of her entwined with penises of various black men.[9] Candy described on her website that she presented photographs of her with various black men, while she was served each week by new, different "cuckold sissies." Candy allowed these cuckolds to prepare her for her black lovers, and required these cuckold servants to also "clean" her afterwards.

An entrepreneur who calls himself "Kingbull" is out to help all the men out there, desperate to get their wives to cuckold them. On the website he sells an eBook, called the "Ultimate Cuckold Manual," an electronic tome that promises to help "wannabe cuckolds" learn how to successfully encourage their wives to pursue sex with other men. Kingbull even offers private chatroom assistance to couples, when you buy his book. Kingbull proposes a new word, "wuckold," combining wittol and cuckold, to describe men who not only tolerate or accept their wife's infidelity, but "thrive on it," and who "enjoys and encourages sexual humiliation, denial and emasculation" from their wife's pursuit of gratification outside their marriage.[10]

He insists that his book will help new cuckolds, whom he calls "nucks," to overcome their wives' objections, and help them to find sexual fulfillment in the arms of other men. Interestingly, he seems to start in pretty reasonable places, encouraging couples to focus on their communication skills, and commanding the husband, above all other things, to listen to his wife. He suggests exercises to help the couple develop their approach to cuckolding, and to prepare for handling safety needs, jealousy, and fears. He encourages couples to role-play together, and helps the husband develop subtle verbal ways to lead his wife slowly into embracing the idea of sex with other men. The author brings in concepts from neurolinguistic programming, a form of subtle, covert hypnotic suggestions. He asserts the importance of these wannabe cucks reassuring their wives that their feelings for their wife won't change, and their relationship will only improve, and become closer. This process "takes time and effort," like any other thing in life, but Kingbull encourages men to stick with it, be patient, and not expect results overnight. He supports the use of basic psychological techniques like shaping, encouraging men to reward and reinforce small steps towards cuckolding, as when their wife flirts with another man. By encouraging one's wife to view that flirting experience as positive, exciting, and allowed, it becomes easier to take her to the next step.

Kingbull asserts that "cuckolding is all about female sexual empowerment, and not just the 'one-handed well-wishing' of the male-dominated fantasy," and that "cuckolding is actually about her sexual liberation." He suggests that "too much of the stuff you find on the Internet" focuses upon the fulfillment of male fantasies, to the exclusion of female desires and interests. Kingbull's book and sales pitch is targeted at men, but he has written it for women as well, including chapters and ideas for women and wives, to help them understand their husband's desires to be cuckolded, and even giving them scripts they can use to more effectively belittle their husbands.

Sage Vivant is a female author and entrepreneur, who took her penchant for writing naughty stories, and turned it into an apparently lucrative business. Sage offered her services online, for hire, penning custom erotica to the request of paying customers. She recently closed this business, in order to return to her own writing, and to "feed my own muse." Her muse led her to publish *Your Erotic Personality: Identifying and Understanding Your Sexual Self.* In this work, Sage offers readers the chance to take interactive quizzes, which help determine what sorts of things turn them on. Then, she offers the reader a variety of erotic personality types, from her experience of catering to the erotic requests of hundreds of customers, writing over a thousand erotic stories. (As an aside there's nothing new about writing erotica for hire. Anais Nin's book *Delta of Venus* is composed of erotic stories that she wrote for an anonymous paying customer, at the price of a dollar a page. She supposedly got this gig from Henry Miller, who had become fatigued with meeting the gentleman patron's erotic needs.) One of the erotic personality types she identifies, is that of the cuckold, which she describes as:

> The Cuckold is turned on by seeing, imagining, or hearing about their lover with somebody else. Cuckolds get hot when they realize they may not be enough to satisfy the seemingly insatiable sexual needs of their lovers—and they may even play a role in finding additional lovers for them to ensure that they get enough sex. They don't get sexually jealous but they do get emotionally attached.[11]

On her website, a cartoon drawing is attached to this description, with a slender white man, standing at a bar, looking over at a woman, presumably his wife, in the arms of a tall black man. Sage discusses the negative connotations often associated with the term cuckold, and suggests that interest in being cuckolded doesn't mean that a man is weak, sexually inadequate, or homosexual. Instead, she suggests that some cuckolds are so confident of their sexual prowess and ability to please a woman that they are not threatened by having and watching someone else sexually pleasure her. She argues that it can make such a man feel very powerful sexually to see that he has a woman who is so strongly driven sexually that she will engage in such wild behavior. That such a sexually alive woman has chosen him for a husband is a source of pride, rather than humiliation.

In a podcast about the cuckold, Sage makes the point that there are female cuckolds out there, and that she has written stories for these women. She also confronts the idea that this is about humiliation. Instead, she asserts that these relationships and fantasies are completely consensual, arranged between the members of a couple, and have far more to do with arousal at the idea of their wife being a "slut, loose woman or harlot." She argues that almost all men have some tendency towards arousal at this idea, and the idea of being with a sexually empowered woman who pursues her own sexual fulfillment. She suggests, though, that cuckolds are those who find this idea the most arousing fantasy. She expects the cuckold fantasy and personality type to gain increasing prominence in times to come, in reflection of the increasing ability to express and pursue this fantasy.

You can take Sage's quiz, and find out your own erotic personality type, at her website.[12] Aside from "the cuckold," other personality types include "the top," "the bottom," "the watcher," "the risk-taker," and many more. Sage suggests that most people have aspects of as many as three or four erotic types, but typically have a "primary" type that is the most arousing for them. When I took the test, I ended up being classified as "a student," who approaches sexuality with the eye of a researcher, who is always looking to learn. How appropriate.

Another enterprising hotwife and her husband have also turned their sexual activities into money online, and not just by posting naked pictures of themselves and other people. At cafepress.com, the hotwife "Naughty Allie" and her husband David sell lingerie, t-shirts, coffee mugs, bumper stickers, and pins, all with a hotwife or cuckold theme. Some of the logos for women's wear say:

> "It's Not Cheating If My Husband Is Watching."
> "Fuck me while my husband watches."
> "I have a husband so let's make this quick."
> "My husband likes to watch."
> "Yes, my husband knows I'm here."[13]

Men and husbands have far less selection in their advertising wear, mainly just "cuckold" and "insignificant other." After all, this is a lifestyle that really is all about the women, from sex to t-shirts.

In Great Britain, a sexual activity called "dogging" carries significant similarities to the casual sex and group sex in hotwifing. According to the BBC, dogging involves couples that drive into secluded areas and have sex in their car, while men outside the car observe, masturbate, often photograph, and sometimes participate. The practice appears to have emerged in the past ten to fifteen years, from the activities of adolescent males, sneaking up and spying on cars where couples, often teenagers themselves, had sex. Some couples ostensibly came to enjoy their admirers, and began leaving the interior light of the car on, during their adventures, to increase their audience's enjoyment. Some couples go further, leaving windows and doors open, inviting and encouraging varying levels of participation, from reaching in and fondling to climbing in the car and "taking a turn." The locations of dogging activities vary, as participants attempt to avoid police and angry neighbors. (Who reportedly purchase and use mobile sirens to drive off the doggers, who flee, thinking the police are on the way.) However, according to current British law, so long as all participants and activities are consensual, and of age, with no "outraged" observers, dogging violates no law.

The Internet and texting via cell phones are used by these couples and bystanders to arrange locations and rendezvous. Dogging spin-offs are now developing, with some individuals practicing "piking," which is sexual arousal as one watches doggers, watching couples. No word yet if there are people that get off watching pikers, who are watching doggers, who are watching couples. Some couples "carp," by posting their cell phone numbers for outside viewers to call, that they might interact safely with their observers, who might then request that the couple in the car engage in activities, or simply move one way or another, to improve their view. As one might imagine, the overwhelming majority of the observers seem to be male, and their pushy, demanding, and intrusive behaviors have, according to some, driven away those couples that are merely looking for light exhibitionism.

The U | Rockers, a British rock band, met while dogging. According to their website, the band members found a common interest, "U | Rockers came together from a chance meeting at a dogging meet in a car park off the M25. They discovered they were all getting off on the music coming from the girl's MX5 as much as they were getting off on watching her and her multiple partners. One thing led to another, and when it was over they found out they were all into making music."[14]

As has been the case with swinging, British officials expressed concern about possible disease transmission, including hepatitis. Whether or not such a connection exists has not been clearly documented or supported, though doggers discuss and acknowledge the need for use of protective measures. A "Newbie's Guide for Doggers" even includes recommendations that doggers have a kit that includes condoms and latex gloves, along with lube, antiseptic wipes, a blanket, and, of course, a flashlight to improve their view.[15] In 2004, Stan Collymore, a famous British soccer player, was caught by two *Sun* reporters while engaged in dogging at a carpark. (No word as to why the reporters were there.) Collymore had a history as a "bad boy" of the sport, and was vilified in the British press in 1998 for striking a girlfriend. (He later attempted to sell a video of himself and this Swedish girlfriend having sex, but the ex-girlfriend put a legal stop to this.) He admitted that he had been dogging for a long time, and had engaged in sex while doing so. As a result of the publicity, he lost his contract as a radio commentator for BBC, but returned to sports broadcasting in 2007, including on BBC. No word if he is still dogging it.

Ashley Lister conducted interviews in Britain of people involved in several different aspects of swinging, including dogging. Eve and Frank were a couple who had been married for five years when they first encountered the thrill of public sex. One night, returning home and more than a little tipsy, Eve performed oral sex on Frank while he drove. At a red light, the driver of a neighboring car expressed his appreciation, to the surprise and excitement of the couple. Aroused by the experience and their audience's reaction, they bypassed their home and drove instead to a nearby dogging spot. There, a dozen men watched while Eve again performed fellatio and masturbated.

> "It was terrifying," Eve said afterwards, "but in a good way. I don't know why people bother themselves with drugs. . . . I can't see the need for heroin or cocaine when you can get so high from a cocktail of sexual excitement and danger."[16]

A week later, they returned, with a "dogging kit," and Eve saying that she now wanted to "touch another man's cock."[17] She performed oral sex through the car window on an onlooker that night, while she lay in the car beneath her husband. When they returned the next week, Eve again upped the ante, now desiring a stranger. In between their visits to dogging sites, the couple's sex life went "ballistic," as they were having sex "like bunnies, talking about what had happened . . . and what we were going to do when we got back there."[18]

Their adventures reached a peak the night Eve decided she wanted Frank to see her with "twelve strangers in one night."[19] At least a dozen strangers crawled into their car their night, having sex with Eve while her husband watched and kissed her. The couple counted the used condoms deposited on the floor of their car that night, and found that Eve had been taken many times that night, by many different men. Eve described to Lister that the encounters were sexually stimulating and even addictive, but that they were also "life-affirming," in that it made her feel attractive, desired, and sexually satisfied to be the object of attention for so many men.[20]

In a news story in the 1990s, the wife of a Florida deputy sheriff was found having sex with various local politicians, while her husband observed and videotaped the proceedings through a mirror built into their closet. This wife, Kathy Willets, defended herself from charges of prostitution, arguing that she was a nymphomaniac and unable to control her sexual desires and behaviors. Out of desperation to satisfy Kathy's sexual needs, her husband began seeking men (as many as eight in a day) to satisfy her. The fact that they recorded the proceedings, and that many prominent, conservative crusading public figures were on video paying Kathy for sex, added to the scandal. The one prominent name released belonged to the vice mayor of Fort Lauderdale, a politician with a conservative stance and a history of crusades against strip clubs.

During trial, Willets and her husband claimed that Kathy was a nymphomaniac, and her husband was impotent, unable to satisfy his wife's insatiable desires. They denied ever charging any of her male lovers, and argued that the men merely left her gifts of cash. They took their arguments even further, claiming that the antidepressant Prozac had supercharged the housewife's libido, to an uncontrollable point. (This was prior to much of the current knowledge that Prozac, and most selective serotonin reuptake inhibitors actually suppress libido and interfere in arousal and orgasm in both males and females. In contrast, the antidepressant buproprion, trade name Welbutrin, does have some documented tendency to increase libido in some recipients.)

Willets went on to recapitulate more of the history of the nymphomania diagnosis, later relabeling herself as a sex-addict, and asserting that her hypersexuality came from low self-esteem, and the need to receive attention and affirmation from these men who came to her for sex.

Kathy Willets was eventually sentenced to community service, and her husband to eighteen months in jail. She went on to tour strip clubs, and star in porno movies, billed as the "Naughty Nympho," or the "Housewife Hooker." At the time of this book, according to the Yahoo! group dedicated to her, she is working as an escort in Las Vegas, Nevada, where an hour of her time costs $1,500. (Her website doesn't mention whether her husband records the hour for posterity, and if there's an additional charge for his services.) At her website she described to her fans that she loves to "insert new members" into her group, and her body.[21] Elsewhere on the Internet, Kathy advertises her prowess even more explicitly, describing her body, her personality, and her style as an escort. She asserted that she is "up for everything," and the more her clients "pop," the more she gets into it.[22]

In September 2006, the wife of the police chief of Snyder, Oklahoma, was "outed" as a "plus-sized nude model" for numerous Internet pornographic websites. Tod Ozmun was an acclaimed leader of the police department, with a history of more drug arrests than any other police chief in the town's history, when residents downloaded nude pictures of his wife Doris, and began distributing them to the town's citizens. As an outcry erupted, with townspeople questioning their police chief's morals, the mayor supported the chief, and Doris released the following statement:

Hi, my name is Doris Ozmun. I am a 43-year-old adult model. I am in no way affiliated with the Snyder Police Department other than the fact I am married to the chief of police, Tod Ozmun. The Web site I am featured on is in no way affiliated with the Snyder Police Department nor the city of Snyder.

I have done nothing illegal, and it is my First Amendment right of the Constitution. You do not have to like or agree with what I do for me to be protected by the First Amendment right.[23]

A few weeks later, the police chief, the mayor, and a Snyder councilman (the councilman reportedly resigned because he did not wish to be associated with the actions of the other city officials) all resigned their positions, "fed up with the public attention" and the incessant demands for the firing of Chief Ozmun. Though attempts had been made to prosecute Doris and the chief, the city council had squashed these efforts, affirming the rights of the First Amendment. Doris later removed the pictures from the Internet, though her husband had earlier told the press, "My wife is 6-foot-3 and weighs 300 pounds. If there is somebody that thinks they can control her, have at it. I have tried for 11 years and haven't been able to."[24]

In March 2008, a Pueblo, Colorado, police officer, Michael Bethel, settled a lawsuit with the city of Pueblo, having alleged that he had been fired for having a cuckold relationship with his wife of twenty years. For the past ten years, Tammy had been allowed to have sex with others, as long as they weren't married or minors, and she told her husband about the encounter. Notably, the arrangement seemed to limit Michael's sexual freedom to only having sex with Tammy, or with others when she was involved.

According to articles in the *Rocky Mountain News*, Bethel was fired for involvement in a complicated issue around a witness's testimony regarding a burglary, where a videotape of Tammy allegedly having sex with the witness was somehow involved.[25] The incident began when Bethel took his wife with him to an apartment, where he had been dispatched as a police monitor as a woman removed her belongings from the apartment of her ex-boyfriend. Bethel later returned to the apartment, allegedly to find a lost notebook. While there, the apartment's resident, the ex-boyfriend, was apparently impressed with Tammy, and invited her to "come back any time." Allegedly, she did, and their sexual encounter was videotaped. It is unclear in the reports whether the encounter involved Michael or not, though it seems that it may have been he that was doing the filming.

As is apparently the destiny of all such videotapes, it was later stolen by the man's ex-girlfriend (the one that moved out, in that first encounter). As the police investigated the case, the video and its contents became known. Michael apparently attempted to prevent the video becoming public but was unsuccessful. He was fired four days later, and charged with witness tampering.

The apartment resident testified against Michael, describing the details of his sexual encounters with Michael and his wife. Michael was not convicted on any charges, and later sued the City of Pueblo in federal court, claiming that he had been wrongfully terminated as a result of the disclosure of his unusual sexual lifestyle. The case was settled, in his favor, for twenty thousand dollars. A photo of Michael and his wife published in the *Rocky Mountain News*, and taken at the conclusion of the long drama, shows Tammy as an extremely attractive Nordic-looking woman with long, straight blonde hair and sharp cheekbones. She was dressed in a long trench coat over what appears to be a corset, revealing a level of cleavage that is probably not often seen in Pueblo courtrooms. No word yet as to whether Mrs. Bethel planned to follow the career path set forth by Mrs. Willets. And what is it, anyway, with police officers and sharing their wives with other men?

It certainly leads me to wonder. Granted, three instances doesn't make a trend, but I have to figure that for every one incident that makes it to the popular press, there were many that were swept under the rug. The only explanation I can really suggest is that this might be an expression of Baumeister's "escapist" theory. Police officers are held to a macho, hypermasculine social expectation. By "giving up" those expectations, allowing and encouraging their wives to sleep with other men, do these police officers receive some respite from the burden of maintaining that invulnerable persona?

The Internet has led to many changes. One of those change is apparent in the content of advice columns. If any man ever wrote to Dear Abby, asking how he could convince his wife to have sex with another man while he watched, the letter was never published. Dan Savage seems to get about a hundred of those letters each week. He has commented that, judging by the letters he receives, there are "legions of men into cuckolding." One wife wrote, complaining that her husband was one of these, and that their relationship had progressed to a point of absolute "incompatibility" as the couple attempted to deal with the impact of the husband's fantasy. Savage suggests to this wife that cuckoldry is "a fetish too far," and that the woman's husband can only ask her to participate, if she is also into it, or at least willing. Savage has used the term "good giving and game" (GGG) to define spouses or partners, who are willing to satisfy their partner's sexual or kinky needs. But, if a wife is not willing to go along, she should be able to say, "You have to drop this. You can fantasize about it whenever you like, but this isn't something I'm ever going to be able to do for you."[26]

Savage has also heard from women who desire to cuckold their husbands, and from gay men who desire to have their husbands cuckold them. Ultimately, however, Savage's patience wears thin with the "legion" of cuckolds and cuckold wannabes who write him, seeking advice on how to encourage their wives to fulfill their fantasies, or whether or not they, the cuckold, are allowed to cheat, when their wife refuses to fulfill their fantasies. Savage has stated that he believes (or hopes) that this is a short-lived phenomenon, popular now only as an Internet-related trend, and soon to die out. Tristan Taormino is a polyamorous and kinky author who occasionally offers guest comments for Dan. She responded to the cuckold issue in Dan's column, highlighting the BDSM elements in the cuckolding fetish, in contrast to Savage's own theories regarding the role of "eroticizing fear" in this sexual practice. She suggested that men may find it enjoyable, to have a "power imbalance," where their wives could sleep with other men, and the husbands did not have a similar sexual feeling.[27] This type of power play can simply serve another role in enhancing sexual arousal.

Technology, by its very nature, opens new doors to new experiences and types of interactions. The Internet is one of the most revolutionary forms of technology in human history, in its creation of social change throughout the world. Like the story of Jamie, in interlude 7, one of the greatest effects of the free exchange of information available on the Internet has been the discovery that people are not alone in their specific, uncommon desires and fantasies. Through the Internet, and powerful search engines, one can now easily find others who share your own interests, and have perhaps taken them further than you have.

KAY AND JOE

*At first, I didn't think I could do it, not being nice. I mean doing
this, being a cuckoldress, it's about not being nice. I found that
I had this inner, secret part of myself that I had always ignored.*

Kay and Joe posted an advertisement on Craigslist, requesting a woman
who would be willing to join them, in "witnessing a cuckold ceremony," to celebrate a "unique relationship." They responded to my e-mail
request for an interview with interest, but asked, "What's in it for us?" I
hadn't gotten such a request before, and with the current state of my bank
account, I wasn't prepared to pay or compensate couples for participating. I had recently received my federal economic stimulus check, and
though it did stir my cockles to envision spending some of that money on
an interview and a topic that would simultaneously "stimulate" and dis-
turb many conservatives, I worried about the precedent that might be set,
if I started paying for interviews. Instead, I offered to buy Joe and Kay dinner, and they readily accepted.

We met at a place that specializes in pastries, coffee, and healthy en-
trees. Interestingly, it turned out to be the place that Kay used to meet and
screen potential "bulls." When they walked up to me, Kay was in front, a
slender redhead, her hair pulled back. She was thirty-six, and wore a black
sweater over her shoulders, jeans, and a white top with a plunging neck-
line. When Kay laughed, often in a rueful, self-reflective way, the muscles
in her neck tensed, showing the tendons in a way that occasionally made
her laughter resemble a painful grimace.

Joe was a stocky, bearded forty-three-year-old man wearing a tan base-
ball cap pulled low over his eyes. While Kay laughed often, Joe was im-
passive, showing very little, if any emotion throughout the interview. He
gradually warmed up, but maintained what seemed to be a customary, in-
nate level of reserve.

While standing in line to order our food, we briefly discussed backgrounds. Kay was from California, near Sacramento, and had moved to New Mexico just a few years before. Joe had lived here his whole life. As we sat down, Joe commented that Joe and Kay were not their real names, but the names they used on the Internet. When signing consent forms, they preferred to sign with initials, rather than reveal their real names. (Given that they offered me assumed names, as I transcribed their interview, I later worried over whether I should change their names again, or use their provided aliases. I worried that in choosing aliases for their aliases, I might accidentally choose their real names. I might worry too much, you think?)

Joe and Kay met through postings on Craigslist. Kay, who had worked as a stripper and exotic dancer for around twelve years, had recently divorced from her second ("and last!" she asserted) marriage. Her first marriage had been to a "self-proclaimed swinger" who liked to watch Kay have sex with lots of men, while he directed the "action." "But," Kay explained, "It was about his fantasies, and about his desires, not mine. I really think that he was using me to fulfill the desires he felt he couldn't fulfill. It was really that he wanted to have sex with those guys himself, but he couldn't bring himself to do it. I could have had more control in it, but then, it was, well, he's the husband; it's about what he wants. Right? But, even after, well, I'm into guys, I get really excited by guys, but I get bored, sort of quick, and want something, someone else. Now, with Joe, I have someone that I love very much, who loves me, who wants to see me have as much pleasure as I can. And, what's wild is that it takes away any feelings of jealousy for me. I can think about Joe being with other women, and it doesn't get me, the way it might have, before we started in cuckolding."

Kay's second marriage ended in jealousy and domestic violence. Craigslist postings were Kay's way of seeking out the "no strings attached, kinky" sexual encounters she wanted. "I've had cookie-cutter relationships, and open relationships. But I wanted to explore, on my terms. I have a slutty side, but I know I have to be careful." Both Joe and Kay acknowledged that with her physical beauty and attributes, she could easily walk into a bar, and ask any random guy "would you like to spank me?" and quickly have a line around the corner of interested males, who were literally chomping at the bit to meet Kay's requests. But, what Kay was looking for was noninvolved sexual encounters with men who would dominate her. Encounters with men who "knew what they were doing," not just men who "were just going along to get in my pants."

It was in this way that they met, with several sexual encounters where Joe dominated Kay. Slowly, they began to talk more, after their sexual encounters, sharing more about their desires and interests. It was after one such encounter, when Kay shared that she intended to "have lots of sex, with lots of different men," that Joe suggested Kay "look up cuckolding." According to the couple, she did, coming back to Joe and saying, "it sounds great, and it sounds like what I want, but what man would ever go along with that? This is all just a fantasy, right? There aren't really guys out there that are into this?"

In fact, there were such men, including Joe, and, gradually, the relationship that began with him in a dominant role began to switch. Joe described that he had always been a "switch," even though this was somewhat frowned upon in "pure" BDSM.

But, Joe had always been interested in both sides, and in going back and forth. When he first made his suggestion to Kay, he didn't have a secret agenda about fulfilling his own interests in cuckoldry. Instead, he merely thought that it was something that might be good for Kay, might help her to become more assertive, and more sexually aggressive. "I've always had a thing for sexually aggressive women. When I grew up, sex was not something that women were supposed to be into. They had sex, or at least, we were told they had sex, once a week, on Wednesdays, with the lights off, doing their duty. But really, at the base, women are just like men, in their sexual desires, but they're told, raised, not to allow that. I find women who reject that, who embrace their sexuality, all of it, aggressively, very, very arousing."

"A lady I worked with in Germany ran a brothel," said Kay. "She did a BDSM male-domination show that I used to see. It was all black leather and whips, and the men cowering on the ground. I thought that was all it was, the black leather, and calling men 'worms' a lot. I thought that was what male domination was, all it was, the black leather, the costumes. When I started learning about cuckoldry, I found it was a lot more than that; there were a lot more options and possibilities. At first, I didn't think I could do it, not being nice. I mean doing this, being a cuckoldress, it's about not being nice. I found that I had this inner, secret part of myself that I had always ignored. I'd never nurtured her. This part of myself that could say things, which under normal circumstances, would hurt somebody's feelings. I found that it turned me on, to explore that. It surprised me, that that was inside me."

As a stripper, Kay could act confidently, and could make men pay attention to her. But, this was always on the outside, and was always an act. Joe described that inside, Kay has always been too nice. "You step on her foot, standing in line; she apologizes to you, for being in your way. She apologizes, or used to, for existing."

Kay was raised in a very strict Christian sect, where her sex, and her sexuality, were both suppressed. She grew up feeling guilty and ashamed of herself, her sex, and growing feelings of sexual desire. Kay recalled that the thing that saved her was when she was babysitting for a couple who had a book about sexual positions. The book also had a section about female ejaculation.

Kay had recently discovered, in her personal sexual explorations, that she squirted during orgasm. Given her complete lack of sexual education, and the absence of any supportive adults from whom she could seek advice and knowledge, Kay had worried that her squirting was abnormal and unhealthy.

"The first time it happened, the first time I had sex, when I was sixteen, I squirted everywhere, all over, all over the bed, the guy I was with. I freaked out, and he did too. He told everybody I peed, peed on him, and the bed, and everything." Kay went on to explain that the book, and later research on her part, had convinced her that female ejaculation was normal, and had opened her eyes to the possibility that her sexuality was potentially positive, and healthy.

"Since we started doing this, and since I moved in with Joe and his wife, I've really started becoming a lot more assertive, a lot more confident about who I am, and really celebrating my sexuality. I'm not ashamed of my sexuality anymore; I love to talk about it. I used to be really sensitive about talking about it, afraid that I would offend somebody. Now, I'm really out there. I found out that I had a secret part of myself that I'd never nurtured. A part of myself that could say something that is not nice. That could say and do things that, under normal circumstances, would hurt somebody's feelings. Surprisingly, I found it was a real turn-on to explore that part of myself. I really get excited, talking about this to my friends. I've got a couple of friends, women, who are like getting excited, converted, they take my stories, my ideas, and go explore them themselves. They can't believe the life I've got, like I've got my cake and get to eat it too they say."

"Women have a lot more power than they know," says Joe. "I really think that this is about empowering women. Women should have a lot more power in our society than they do. But I also think that women need to acknowledge that there are different ways of living, that the 'white picket fence fantasy' is just that, a fantasy."

"I can be bi, sometimes, with the right woman, in the right situation. I admire a woman's body, especially when it's really hot, but basically, I'm pretty straight. I like [men], I just want a lot of it, a lot more than just one," laughed Kay.

"I can admire a guy's body," agreed Joe. "I used to work out a lot, in the gym all the time, and I can admire when a guy's body is in shape, but I just don't think the male body has the beauty of a female figure. But, I guess I can be considered 'orally submissive.' When we're fantasizing together, during sex, sometimes we fantasize about what it would be like, with a guy, for me to be forced to go down on him."

Excitedly, Kay jumps in, "It's such an incredible turn on for me, to have that kind of power. My first husband wanted me to dominate him, to tie him up, in black leather, etc. But, I couldn't do that. I can't really dominate someone that I don't respect. But now, with Joe, and envisioning myself, forcing two guys to do whatever I want, to satisfy me, my desires, I'm in control. Really, the idea of two guys having sex with each other doesn't actually turn me on. But, taking two straight, hot guys, that are at my control, and forcing them to do something, with each other that is just so, absolutely against their nature." Kay literally shivered, with a physical chill of excitement at the thought. "Even if, especially if, the guys aren't bi at all, forcing them to do that is just an incredible thrill. I'm into guys that are not metrosexual at all, guys that are real men, really comfortable in their own skin, who would never, ever be with another guy. And the ideas of making them do that, wow. It really, really gets me going."

Curious, I ask Joe and Kay to tell me more about the kinds of men they choose. Joe told me that they get an unbelievable number of responses to Craigslist ads, and even more when the men find out how attractive Kay is. But, many of the men are not appealing. Joe went on to reveal that a lot of the people in cuckolding are really into what he calls "BBC. Big Black Cock. It's really offensive to me. I think it's just really, really blatant racism."

Kay added her own thoughts, "I want attractive guys. Since this is my fantasy, I think I can be selective. It's my fantasy, so I can have the prettiest piece of meat behind the counter. I want bulls, men who are going to be respectful. Bulls that recognize that I'm in charge of this whole situation. They have to understand how this works, that can get into the mind-set of it. A lot of them think it's just about getting some. They come in and think that they're supposed to just order my husband and I around. But really, it's about me getting off. I tell them, you'll come in, we'll do our thing, you'll get off, and then it's time for you to go. Leave."

The couple has arranged things with mirrors, so Joe can observe. For some men, the situation is intimidating, and some men have been unable to sexually perform under the pressure. Joe can see Kay's face during the sexual encounter, and said that that is all he wants to see, to see her enjoying herself with another man. Afterwards, when the other man leaves, the couple has intense sex. Kay taunts Joe, humiliating him, and sometimes even "rubbing his face in It." Kay described how her adrenaline rushes as she explores the power of being in charge over Joe. In the six months that the couple have been living together, they have acted out this scene about five or six times, and find that the sexual excitement both before and after the actual event is a tremendous sexual thrill.

The table had, by now, been cleared, and the restaurant is nearly empty. Workers had brought the patio furniture inside, and it was clear that we are only a short time from being asked to leave. Surprisingly, our dinner conversation had not caused any attention. As we talked, I noticed that both Joe and Kay were conscious and aware of the people around them, occasionally dropping their voices so people couldn't hear. Both seemed to be very aware of any children that came around the table, and we were lucky, I suppose, that no families chose to sit near us.

I reminded them of the advertisement they posted, requesting a female to witness a "cuckold ceremony." What did they mean? What sort of ceremony did they envision?

"It was pretty impulsive, really. We post lots of ads, just to see what and who is out there," Joe says. "I love the Internet. I'm on it a lot. There's so much freedom now because of it. Now, we can post ads, and find people out there, that are like us. I think that's why there's been such an explosion of cuckold stuff. People were always into it, but now they can find out they're not the only ones. There is a lot of this around. Kay asked at a bar once, the bartender, and the people at the bar. Most of the guys knew about this, knew what cuckolding was. None of the women did."

"I kind of had a vision of another woman, and the two of us dominating Joe together. He and I fantasize about that sometimes, having two women, two cuckoldresses, both of us dominating Joe."

Our interview ended, shortly before they turned off the lights in the restaurant. For all the nonchalance that Joe and Kay showed, they seemed eager to talk about their lifestyle, as were so many other couples. Joe shared, that while Kay talked about their lifestyle with her friends, he had no one that he could discuss these things with, in real life, apart from the Internet.

10

FECUND FLUIDS

So they stood in the utter, dark kiss, that triumphed over them
both, subjected them, knitted them into one fecund nucleus of the
fluid darkness.

D. H. Lawrence[1]

Evolutionary researchers now suggest that human sexuality evolved
and developed with an expectation, or at least acceptance of the risk,
of female sexual infidelity. Cuckoldry could upset the apple cart, and
lead a man to invest in children to whom he had no genetic relationship.
And so, like the Russians and the Americans during the Cold War, an
arms race began, with male and female sexual adaptations developing,
which affected the fertilization process, and combated the effects of the
other sexes adaptations. Much of this quiet battle for dominance is
played out amongst the moist fluids of the human body, the fecund wet-
lands of the genitals and the brain.

The story of female ejaculation is a complex one, embroiled in the see-
sawing arguments over whether vaginal or clitoral orgasms reign. Freud
mentioned "abnormal vaginal secretions" as a source of female disgust.
Historically, female ejaculation has been acknowledged, sometimes in
celebration, and sometimes in shame. "Female fecund fluids," "female
semen," and ejaculations of the "female prostate" have all described this
phenomenon, where an excited woman, as Kay described in our interview, "soaks the bed." Psychologist Josephine Lowndes Sevely reviews

and celebrates much of this history in *Eve's Secrets, a New Theory of Female Sexuality*.[2] From Hippocrates, who argued that male and female ejaculatory fluids combined to create life, to Freud, who condemned such a response as evidence of "immature" sexuality and personality development, this female response has generated controversy but surprisingly little developed research.

The ancient Greeks celebrated female sexual fluids as "generative," and involved in not only sexual pleasure but also in the very creation of life itself. The Hebrews distinguished female sexual fluids from the "unclean" menstrual fluids. Contact with menstrual fluids generated prohibitions as described in the texts of Leviticus where menstruating women are to be isolated from others, and any man who contacts menstrual fluid is likewise banished and isolated. Female sexual fluids generate no such prohibitions.

Lowndes Sevely cites references to female ejaculation, found in American Indians, and Pacific Islanders, though it was sometimes mistaken for urination, but was clearly linked to the female's sexual pleasure. Hindu and Tantric texts identify female ejaculation as linked to the "great pleasure" of the female, and note that it requires far more time and stimulation to achieve than does male ejaculation.

In the days of vulvular stimulation, when doctors used manual, and sometimes mechanical massage to trigger "hysterical paroxysms" in their female patients, there was much debate over whether it was ethical or healthy to cause the female to "expel seed." Some doctors held that retention of female seed could cause illness or madness, and it was thus a doctor's duty to assist in relieving this condition.

Though Kinsey acknowledged the existence of female ejaculation, he did not connect this with orgasm. Masters and Johnson likewise described how female orgasm was like males, though without ejaculation. Though female subjects described the expulsion of fluids, these researchers believed that female ejaculation was not connected with female orgasm, and was likely a rare, incidental phenomenon.

Much of the controversy around female ejaculation involves concerns over what the ejaculate actually consists of. Is it urine or not? Are these women merely "peeing the bed," as Kay's teenage lover accused her, or are these fluids emerging from different biological processes? To some degree, scientific controversy and disagreement persist on this front. Some studies of female ejaculation show conclusively that these fluids are not urine. They include mucus fluids, secretions from urogenital glands, including sweat glands. Female ejaculate contains very little urea—far, far less than is found in urine. Other studies, cited by Masters and Johnson, report that studies of female ejaculate are indistinguishable from urine. In fact, Masters and Johnson go so far as to blame female ejaculation on bladder and genital dysfunctions, such as incontinence.

Ejaculatory fluids in the female are expelled through many different ducts in the urethra, often in spurts or jets. During heterosexual intercourse, the penis, and physical pressure, leads to these fluids being expelled into the vagina itself. Recent research also suggests that in many women who do not exhibit noticeable external female ejaculation, the prostatic fluid is actually shunted into the female bladder, in a process similar to what is known as retrograde ejaculation in males.

Glands in the urogenital tract, now called the "Skene's Glands," have been identified as having a pivotal role and appear to serve as a "female prostate," generating sexually related fluids in females, similar to the manner in which the prostate in males generates seminal fluid, in which sperm is delivered. Whether or not the Skene's glands are physiologically sensitive to physical stimulation, as is apparently involved in female ejaculation and orgasm, remains in question.

The G-spot, named after the German gynecologist Ernst Grafenberg, was described and written about in the 1980s. The concept was embraced by the public and by sexuality professionals, but remains controversial and disputed in the scientific community, even to this day. A study published in 2008 by Italian researchers suggests that ultrasound scans of women reveal that those reporting "vaginal orgasms" have areas of thicker tissue in an area of the vagina. Previous reports of similar findings remain controversial, over whether there are not enough nerve endings in that tissue, to play a role in sexual stimulation. However, research has shown that the arrangement, location, and size of glands within the female vagina vary significantly between women. This appears to play a role in the variability and continuing ambiguity regarding both the presence of the G-spot, and the phenomenon of female ejaculation.

Lisa Lawless, a psychotherapist who earned a doctorate in sexology, has made a career and profession of teaching female ejaculation. She has produced videos and books that support the idea that all women can experience female ejaculation, and that those who do not may be missing something extraordinary. Her website describes much of the history and controversy over female ejaculation, offers links to her books and videos, and to sex toys that she suggests can assist in achieving female ejaculation.[3] Dr. Lawless suggests that female ejaculation may actually improve female urogenital health, in a manner similar to the supposed health aspects of male prostate massage. However, one must note that prostate massage is not currently used in a medically endorsed fashion to treat any conditions, and may even result in some significant medical and health complications such as blood poisoning and even aggravation of prostate cancer.

How many women experience ejaculation is unknown. (One survey suggests around 40 percent.) Some writers believe that all women have the ability to ejaculate, and that achieving this heightens and increases their sexual arousal. Given the variability in the female glands in the vagina, it does seem that a universal female capacity for ejaculation is unlikely. For most women, female ejaculation occurs following one or two "normal orgasms." Women report that female ejaculation occurs following internal stimulation, and particularly manual stimulation of the "G-spot," where many glands appear to be located. Subsequent orgasm, following this stimulation, appears to trigger the expulsion of the fluids generated by these glands.

Because the prostatic fluids typically expelled during female ejaculation are distinct from the slippery mucus and lubricatory fluids more commonly observed in the vagina, the biological role of these fluids is in some question. In the male, prostatic fluids provide a fluid environment, along with nutrients, for sperm. In females, these prostatic fluids may serve some role in cleansing the vagina, assisting in the shedding of dead cells, and maintaining the necessary ph balance in the vaginal environment. Also, while female ejaculation is often linked with female orgasm, research has shown that it is not universally connected to the orgasm, and sometimes occurs independently, both before and after the orgasm, as well as coincidental with the orgasm. It is speculated that female ejaculation may serve an evolutionary process, cleansing or flushing the vagina of semen. The female reproductive system has a number of different physiological strategies that increase the ability of the female to "select" the male by whom she may be fertilized, out of multiple males with whom she has genital intercourse. Through the flushing action, female ejaculation may cleanse the vagina of semen, increasing the likelihood of fertilization by a subsequent male.

I suspect that this controversy, and the resistance by researchers such as Masters and Johnson to acknowledge female ejaculation, and the existence of the G-spot, has to do with the hard-fought battle waged against the idea of the "vaginal orgasm." To acknowledge the role of female ejaculation and the G-spot, may seem to endanger the victories won with the "clitoral orgasm," and might lead to conceivable return to the days where the clitoral orgasm is seen as "less," or even "immature." This approach led to guilt, shame, and sexual problems in the past, for many women, and could renew and prolong a future cycle of social and clinical perspectives that inhibit and suppress female sexuality.

The arguments that integrate clitoral orgasms and G-spot/female ejaculations, and treat female sexuality in a more holistic, comprehensive manner, ultimately strike me as the views most likely to effectively resolve these issues. When there are women that can experience orgasm from having their ears nibbled, or their lower back stimulated, the argument must be broadened. (Sexual research with spinal cord-injured patients, both male and female, has shown a remarkable diversity in physical stimulation that can trigger an orgasm. Physiological monitoring has shown that the individual's response is indistinguishable from a genitally produced orgasm, even when it is triggered by, for instance, stroking of the individual's knee. Kinsey reported on some individuals reportedly able to have an orgasm from similar stimulation, even with intact spinal cords.) Sexual arousal, response, and orgasm involve far more than one small part of the genitals, especially in women.

Female orgasm, particularly multiple female orgasms, may work on a principle of "upsucking," such that it increases the likelihood of fertilization, by drawing into the cervix increased amounts of sperm, through the muscular and tissue contractions and pulses of orgasm. Further, it may actually give a woman's body some control of whose sperm is most likely to fertilize her eggs, if she exerts control over her orgasm, and which male partner she experiences it with. Some theorists have suggested that the female orgasm (and the contents of semen) might have evolved to increase the likelihood that a woman will remain reclining after sex, and reduce the likelihood of the sperm being drawn out of the vagina by gravity.

Female orgasm serves other purposes, in terms of mating strategies. As my wife has commented, a woman who finds a man with whom she is more orgasmic is more likely to stay with that man, given the choice.

This is called the "Mister Right" hypothesis. However, the evidence showing that many women engaging in extramarital sex report that they are more orgasmic with men other than their husband subtly contrasts with this theory.

A woman experiencing orgasm with her husband might also send a reassuring message to that husband, that he has sexually satisfied his wife, and that he doesn't need to worry about her seeking sexual satisfaction with other men.

Women more frequently fake orgasms than men, and, women are more likely to fake orgasms when with their long-term mate, than when they are in short-term sexual relationships. Far more women call into sexual advice radio and television shows, complaining that their husband is "too quiet" during sex, compared to men. Women, by and large, appear to be far more vocal during orgasm and sex than men. Studies of chimpanzees show that female chimps are more vocal during sex when there are other males around, but are quieter when other females are around. One suggestion to explain this is that females may be seeking to attract other males, for additional mating opportunities, and to thus increase the chances of sperm competition ensuring that the female gets impregnated with "winner" sperm. Females might be quiet when other females are around in order to reduce the chances that the male might choose to be with another female, if one were to make herself available. Victorian marriage manuals counseled women that their orgasm and sexual responsiveness must be tempered and restrained, lest they lead their husbands to fear that their wife was so sexually driven that she might seek, or succumb to, sex outside their marriage. Thus, the response of a husband to his wife's orgasm could truly go in almost any direction. A study of mating habits of African primates found that when the female macaque was more vocal, the male was more likely (59 percent) to ejaculate during intercourse with that female. Quiet females had far less success in inducing orgasm in the males.

Regardless of female orgasm, the anatomy of the vagina retains sperm following sexual intercourse. While there is what is called "flowback," where fluid and semen drip from a woman's vagina after sex, this flowback often does not occur for some time after intercourse, sometimes as long as thirty minutes. This is due to the formation of a pool, or a cup, within the vagina, near the cervix, where the sperm collects. There may be some immediate discharge of semen (in zebras, there is an immediate, dramatically expulsive fountain of sperm that the female ejects from her vagina), but much of the semen is collected in this pool, from which it is then transported by the anatomy of the vagina and cervix, up to the woman's womb.

Female orgasm leads to the shedding of some internal cells and fluids, which carry away some sperm, and clears passages in a woman's cervix. In this fashion, a woman might rid her cervix of the sperm that is already within her, typically from her husband or mate. Because this sperm is the sperm that has been "topped off" by the man, it is often older, "blocker" sperm. Thus, a woman's orgasm appears to "open the doors" to the seed of her lover, increasing the chance of fertilization by him, even with the sperm of her mate still within her vagina.

Second, the woman's orgasm increases the overall retention of a lover's sperm. When a female has an orgasm during heterosexual, unprotected intercourse, studies indicate that as much as 70 percent of her lover's sperm is retained within her vagina and cervix. In contrast, without orgasm only about 30 percent is retained. This occurs, in part, due to the fact that the female orgasm weakens the cervical mucus filter, creating more channels for sperm to reach the womb, and the muscular contractions of the vagina in orgasm actually "suck" more sperm up into the cervix. Thus, this suggests that males who are able to induce female orgasm more adeptly are more likely to be reproductively successful.

In a large British study that examined both menstrual cycles and the sexual activity of women, women engaged in infidelity tended to have sex with their lovers, rather than their husbands, more often when they were most fertile (recall that this is also the time when women at nightclubs are most likely to dress in a revealing fashion). These women also used birth control methods less consistently, during their ovulatory periods. Other studies have shown that among married women, there is an increase in sexual fantasies about men other than their husbands, and greater feelings of attraction to other men, as the women approach more fertile periods of their cycles. Women who are engaged in infidelity report that they have almost three times as many orgasms in a week, compared to those who are monogamous.

During the Middle Ages, a common European belief was that swallowing a man's semen promised to make the man "burn" with love for the woman. In contrast, current research suggests that swallowing semen might have more physiological impact upon the swallower than the, umm, swallowee. Psychology researchers at SUNY in Albany published a study of depression in sexually active female college students. What this data suggested was that female students who had sex without a condom reported less depression than either women who used condoms, or those who didn't have sex at all. The authors speculated in their 2002 paper that semen might have an antidepressant quality for women. The lead author, Gordon Gallup, suggested that these effects might have an evolutionarily driven role by improving the bonds between a couple. Gallup also noted that their research also indicated that semen helped alleviate menstrual discomfort in the women who did not use condoms.

Researchers Gallup and Rebecca Burch didn't stop there. Their results sparked a whole range of studies, as they began to examine the other potential effects of semen—physiological and behavioral—upon the human body. (Note, I didn't say female; the researchers included consideration of the effect of semen upon men, when received during oral or anal sex.) The list of semen components and their potential effects reads like a health food ingredient list. A time may come when men are required by the FDA to have this list tattooed near their genitals. The below list is only a partial one, and the research continues. According to the summary of research by Gallup and Burch, semen often contains the following chemical and hormonal components, which might result in the following effects:

- Testosterone—When administered through the vagina or anus, testosterone is absorbed at higher rates than when administered through the skin as a cream (the typical means of medical administration). Testosterone can increase libido in both men and women, though the role of testosterone in female libido remains somewhat ambiguous.
- Estrogen, dopamine, and other hormones are present in semen, all of which have some noted impact upon increasing a female's interest in sexual activity.
- Prostaglandins in semen may actually trigger or induce menstruation in some cases. While this seems self-defeating, these hormones might trigger either release of the female ova, making it available for fertilization, or trigger menstruation, in order to prevent fertilization by other men, essentially clearing the playing field. Prostaglandin

also suppresses a woman's immune response, helping the man's sperm to survive attack by the woman's immune system.

- Epinephrine, norepinephrine, oxytocin, vasopressin, melatonin, and other opioids are all present in semen, and all have detectable impact upon cognition and memory. Burch and Gallup found that semen appeared to reduce depression in women; it also improved their ability to make effective, quick decisions and improved their concentration. The improvement of memory might serve to help women create stable memories of their sexual encounter. (Let's just hope they're good memories—that is still apparently up to the male partners.)

- Melatonin in semen may also increase sleepiness, and oxytocin can encourage bonding and attachment behaviors such as cuddling. Both of these effects can serve to increase the time that a woman spends in a reclining or supine position after sex, increasing the chances that a man's sperm can reach her cervix and thence her eggs.

- Cortisol in semen may serve to create a feeling of pleasure in a woman, reinforcing the act of sex and making it more likely the woman will repeat the behavior.

- Luteinizing hormone is present in semen at five times the rate that it is present in blood, and serves to stimulate the release and maturation of the female egg, increasing the chances of fertilization. Other hormones normally associated with the female placenta, such as gonadotropin are also present in semen at very high levels, and may support successful conception and implantation of an embryo.

- Oxytocin present in semen may reduce the incidence of preeclampsia in pregnant women, especially when it is ingested during oral sex.

- Estrogen, serotonin, endorphins, and other neurotransmitters are present in semen at levels that may effect the levels of and feelings of depression in both males and females. These same hormones may also serve to modulate the effects of postpartum depression, menopausal depression, and premenstrual syndrome. Indeed, Burch and Gallup even suggest that some of the symptoms associated with these syndromes might actually reflect withdrawal from the positive effects of semen, as the negative impact of these syndromes is reduced when couples continue sexual activity on a regular, frequent basis.[4]

Many of these effects seem awfully theoretical and speculative and are based upon potential effects of sometimes minute quantities of these various compounds in semen. However, a growing body of research suggests that characteristics of semen not directly related to fertilization have played vital roles in the evolution of human sexuality, as males try to increase the chances that their semen will have a chance at fertilizing the woman, either now, or in the future. In other words, male ejaculation has been a weapon in the battle between males and females to control the reproductive outcomes of sexual behavior. There are, of course, remaining questions in this research and further studies to determine whether such small amounts of hormones and substances can generate behavioral or psychological changes. But, this line of research is a fascinating insight into many sexual problems, issues, and oddities.

Whether these effects have any causal link to female promiscuity remains to be seen. But, there is a fascinating series of parallels between the potential effects of the chemicals and hormones within semen, and the behaviors of some women. Regardless of the response of a woman's body to sexual intercourse, a man's semen contains sperm that are organized with a sophisticated, responsive strategy for battle.

Robin Baker and Mark Bellis have led much of the research investigating the sophisticated biological mechanisms and strategies employed by both males and females in their reproductive efforts. The fascinating thing about their arguments is that the behaviors and strategies they explore occur at invisible physiological levels within the bodies of the men and women. In what Baker calls "sperm wars," there are behavioral and biological mechanisms employed to exert control over whose sperm is most likely to fertilize the woman's ovum. Because the female period of fertility and ovulation is hidden in humans, male strategies for fertilization must be more varied than they are in species where the female period of ovulation is more overt. (Like when a cat is in heat—you know it. The entire household and neighborhood knows it too.)

Accepting the premise that humans evolved in a promiscuous, nonmonogamous environment, where a man's sperm had to "compete" with the sperm of other men in a woman's vagina, Baker and Bellis suggest that the process of natural selection acted upon the physiology of males, females, sperm, eggs, and all the reproductive parts involved in procreation. In addition to the size and shape of the penis and testicles, they suggest this process acted upon the nature and function of sperm.

A central piece of their premise is based upon the physiology of sperm. In contrast to the female ova, which a woman is born with, sperm have a very short lifespan, though "shelf life" is perhaps a more accurate term. Sperm last for a few weeks or so, within a male's body. Within a female's vagina and cervix, sperm are most efficacious around three days after being ejaculated into the female's body. "Fresher" sperm are able to be more active, faster, and more motile, for longer periods of time, after ejaculation. Younger sperm are not only more "able" in their efforts to reach and fertilize the female's ovum, but are also more able to actually combat another male's sperm. Fresher sperm contain more of what the researchers call "killer" sperm, which actually have caps that contain fluids that will dissolve other sperm. However, these killer sperm attack only the sperm of another male.

Older sperm use a different strategy. Older sperm do not attack, but instead "block" the sperm of other males from gaining access to the ovum. In the female reproductive system, sperm don't actually "swim" the whole way to the egg. Instead, channels in the cervix, and mucus within these channels work to transport the sperm to the womb and the egg like amphibious vehicles transporting soldiers to the beach at Normandy. The blocker sperm, like the killer sperm, "recognize their own," and allow only their brethren to pass, as they fill up the channels and prevent access by another man's sperm.

Sometimes, the sperm even work together, like teams, rather than individual soldiers. Recent research at the University of Sheffield in England has found continuing evidence of changes in sperm physiology and behavior, in response to female promiscuity. The sperm of some rodents develop hook-shaped heads, allowing the sperm to link their hooks, and plow forward through the masses of sperm from other males. Like people linking arms to force their way forward through a concert crowd, the sperm display this physiological adaptation, and behavior, only in rodents where the females are intensely promiscuous.

In a mated couple, the male and his sperm fill the woman's cervix with blocker sperm. It takes somewhere around two to three days for sperm to reach the point at which they can most effectively fertilize an egg. The sperm's shelf life is around five days. Thus, Baker and Bellis suggest that the sperm from the male of a mated couple will typically work to top off the woman's cervix, filling the cervical channels and keeping them filled by replacing expired sperm. In a monogamous couple, the male typically produces smaller numbers of sperm during intercourse; often just enough to add to his wife's gas tank, bringing that needle back up to "F."

When a man has sex with his mate, the numbers of sperm produced is tied to the chances that the female may have had even a chance of sexual encounter with another male. Studies have shown that when a couple is together constantly, the male produces fewer sperm, and greater numbers of sperm are produced when the female is "out of his sight."

When a man has intercourse with a woman who is not his mate, he tends to produce more sperm that is more active and aggressive. This is accomplished in a few ways. When a male masturbates, he ejaculates fewer sperm than he does during intercourse. But, the sperm he does ejaculate after masturbation are older sperm that are less vital. A similar effect is achieved after a nocturnal emission. Both behaviors seem to be male methods that increase the chance of a man's sperm "winning the sperm war." Similarly, when a man ejaculates more than once during a sexual encounter, later ejaculations are more likely to contain "fresher" sperm.

Robin Baker suggests that sperm warfare is not merely a fact of human evolutionary past, but is still acting upon human reproduction today. He cites studies that suggest that as many as 4 percent of children born in Britain today are born from "sperm warfare," where the sperm of different males competed in the mother's vagina. Baker further argues that research indicates that most people living in the modern world have recent ancestors who were born as a result of competing sperm.

In Uri Wernik's research, he found a surprising number of men who eroticized semen, particularly the semen of other men. These men found the presence of another man's semen in or on their wife to be an extremely stimulating and powerful image, and several also commented on the idea of there being the sperm of two men, mixed-up in the wife's body. Many of the men interviewed in this book also eroticized the semen of other men, commenting on it as a powerful visual and tactile symbol of their wife's sexual connection with another man. These husbands discussed as well the tactile feeling of penetrating their wife's vagina (the "silky feeling" referenced by Andrew, in interlude 1), after another man had ejaculated within her, and attributed significant emotional impact to this experience.

One man described the adventures he and his wife have had with the semen of other men. They have arranged unprotected sexual encounters with other men, after medical testing, as his wife doesn't feel truly "taken" until she has the semen of a man either on or in her. Her excitement is enhanced by having the semen of more than one man in her at the same time. With three other couples, they arranged a "bareback gangbang," with six men who underwent testing. The various wives competed with each other, each egging the other on to greater heights of sexual indulgence, reveling in the sensation of multiple men ejaculating in and on them. And their husbands learned to enjoy the sensations of their wives filled with the semen of other men.[5]

Among the Romans, where women were forbidden to drink wine, husbands would sometimes kiss their wives to detect the taste of wine in her mouth. Similarly, it has been suggested that oral sex might have developed as a strategy to detect evidence of sexual infidelity. Many cuckold fetishists and hotwife husbands take this anticuckoldry mechanism and turn it on it's head, fantasizing about the "creampie," performing oral sex on their wife, while her vagina contains the ejaculate of another man, and literally consuming that ejaculate.

A danger in evolutionary theories is the ease with which such "Just So" stories can be created. Just So stories were stories written by Rudyard Kipling to explain such things as how the leopard got his spots, or how the armadillo was created through the mating of a hedgehog and a turtle. Just because an explanatory story can be developed, using the theories and motivations of evolution and natural selection, does not make that story or explanation factual, scientific, or even particularly likely. Those men and women who celebrate "creampies" in their sexuality describe nothing about such motivations, but instead described the sensuality of dominance, bisexuality, and the clear evidence of their wife's sexual contact with another man.

In *The Mammoth Book of Women's Erotic Fantasies*, by Sonia Florens, a contributor from Nottingham, Britain, described her fantasies in a segment called "Cuckold Heaven."[6] In it, the contributor fantasized about aggressively pursuing sex with men other than her "nice" and "grateful" husband, and finding a man who would respond to her aggression in kind. She fantasized about returning home with the evidence of her infidelity, and forcing her husband to clean her with his tongue. She described that her fantasies were one of her only ways to escape her "drab, middle-class housewife and mother's existence." Evolutionary theorists could easily go on to describe how the sexual arousal of such things emerges from the evolutionary underpinnings, but sometimes, I think one has to stop with what someone describes as their motivations.

Likewise, the cuckoldress practice of prohibiting masturbation could, in the theories of Baker, be driven by the female's desire to limit the effectiveness of the husband's sperm, and increase the likelihood of fertilization by another male lover. Prevention of masturbation increases the chances that the husband's sperm will be older, less active, and less able to combat the sperm of a more "virile" male. The older sperm of the husband is thus more suited to a "blocking" strategy. But, with the other lover's sperm already placed, and being transferred up to the cervix and the womb, a blocking strategy is extremely unlikely to be effective. But, the aspects of dominance, and sexual control, of withholding and increasing anticipation, while they may have evolutionary underpinnings, may also simply point to the experiences in this practice which the practitioners find arousing, erotic, and stimulating.

It is likely that it is not only the fluids of the genitals that are involved in the excitement and stimulation experienced by couples who pursue wife sharing. The fluids and chemicals within the brain may play an even greater role, in affecting their choices, their behaviors, and their passion for each other, and their passion for the wife having sex with other men.

> Couples wishing to overcome the boredom of their marital bedrooms, while preserving their marriages, could become eroticized by contact with other people at Sandstone, and later they could divert this sexual energy back into their own relationships . . . while women, particularly those who had been monogamous in long-term marriages, could reexperience with a new man old feelings of being desired, sexually free, unaccountable—indeed many couples could relive during evenings at Sandstone, in ways that were not always harmonious to their marriages, but were individually regenerative, the élan of youthful courtship. [7]

In 1974, researchers Donald Dutton and Arthur Aron used the Capilano Canyon Suspension Bridge in Vancouver to investigate the role of excitement and arousal in the formation of relationships, and sexual imagery. The bridge is 5 feet wide, 450 feet long, and is made of wooden boards attached to wire cables that span a height of 250 feet. When research subjects crossed the bridge and then wrote a story as part of the study, their stories contained far more sexual images and references than stories generated by subjects who did not cross the bridge. Research subjects also developed significant feelings of attraction for a female research assistant, and described feeling "lovestruck," when they encountered the female assistant after crossing the bridge. This research generated theories that have been consistently supported which suggest that when two people of opposite sex do something exciting or physically risky together, it stimulates feelings of sexual attraction and arousal. Recent studies have added further understanding of this phenomenon, and suggest that when two people are not in a sexual or intimate relationship and do something like riding a roller coaster, the experience increases their feelings of sexual attraction and interest in the other person. Notably, though, a roller coaster ride together does not increase feelings of attractedness between a couple, when the two people are already in an intimate relationship. Dr. Daniel Amen, a neuroscientist and psychiatrist, suggests in his book *Sex on the Brain* that couples who have experienced loss of excitement and novelty in their relationships can jump-start their relationships by doing things like skydiving together. Unfortunately, these research studies suggest that while these experiences might stimulate brain neurochemistry, they are unlikely to lead to a renewed or increased feeling of sexual attraction or trigger increased sexual arousal.

> Considering that a big part of cuckolding is the idea of having to have another man please your wife because of a lack of size or whatever excuse real or imagined on the husband's part includes a bit of humiliation. Having your wife with a black man is just ramping up that humiliation because of the taboo factor. If your wife and her [other man] like to go out for dinner or dancing, not many people will really notice if she is out with a white guy but a sexy woman being openly affectionate with a black man well that will get attention. So I think the attraction is the taboo. This lifestyle already breaks with the traditional. Having a black lover just takes it that much further.[8]

The excitement of just "pushing the limits," and engaging in something that is so socially taboo and forbidden is, in and of itself, a motivator for some of these couples' practices. In the activities of Leopold von Sacher-Masoch, the taboo and forbidden nature of being made a cuckold was the thrill. Some cuckolded husbands identify clearly that it is the "extreme" nature of this sexual behavior that drives some of their excitement. On the OurHotwives.org site, contributors shared:

> I actually like that cuckolding—to the extent it's acknowledged at all— is seen as so aberrant, rare and inexplicable. I think it's different from being "taboo" since it describes something few people are aware of! I'm not sure I agree with the presumption that all our passion for this is grounded in jealousy. There are a lot of emotions I feel about my wife making love to other men, but I can't say that raw jealousy is among them.[9]

> Speaking for myself . . . I think the biggest thing for me was the "taboo" factor. It's kind of like lesbian porn. It doesn't do anything for me. Why? Well . . . they don't find it taboo; it's a natural thing for them. Oh, but . . . to watch some straight girl being seduced by another girl . . . deliciously hot. Why do I not want to see my fiance's lover alone? Why do I only want to suck his cock in front of her? If I start seeing him outside the context of her cuckolding me by being with him . . . it's gay sex and that doesn't really do anything for me. I think the same applies to the interracial fetish for many cuckolds. "Society says" (cue the dark, ominous music) it shouldn't be (tsk-tsk), so we're bad little boys and girls for engaging in such foolishness.[10]

Some researchers have suggested that one shouldn't have sex with people you don't love because you'll end up falling in love with them due to the chemistry that happens in the brain during sex with another person. Linda Wolfe wrote in 1975 that this risk was inherent in experimental marriages, in that the tendency to attach to a sexual partner was subtle enough that many people ended up developing intense attachments before they realized the bond was forming. Part of the subtle nature of the bonds that form during sex has to do with the underlying biological mechanics of the brain.

Influential in the human brain during sex and love is the neurochemical phenylethylamine (PEA), also found at small levels in chocolate. This chemical floods the brain when we first fall in love, and works to speed up the information exchange in nerve cells of the brain. This chemical, along with dopamine and serotonin lead to the feelings of euphoria and "walking on air" that we feel when we first fall in love. (No wonder we buy chocolate for our love interests!)

In many animals and humans, a neurochemical called oxytocin appears highly involved in the early phases of intimate sexual relationships. When the amount of oxytocin is increased in a small rodent called a prairie vole, sexual promiscuity increases as well. In humans, oxytocin triggers uterine contractions during birth. Pitocin, used to artificially induce labor, is a chemical analogue to oxytocin.

Oxytocin also does some other remarkable things in the brain. It leads to an amnesic effect, blocking negative memories people have. In other words, it may allow you to be sexually aroused with someone that you were pissed off with, half an hour ago, by "turning off" those memories (make-up sex?). Oxytocin makes the skin more sensitive to touch, heightening the physical sensations experienced during sexual contact. In women, the higher the levels of natural oxytocin in the blood, the more intense their orgasms are. Oxytocin also makes people more trusting, as was demonstrated in an experiment where people inhaled oxytocin, then played an investment game. Oxytocin made participants more likely to give more money for chancy returns to their partners in the game. Higher levels of oxytocin increase fertility, by decreasing chemicals that inhibit conception.

The role of oxytocin can easily be misunderstood, and twisted to fit whatever argument one might wish to make. In 2006, the deputy assistant secretary of the U.S. Department of Health and Human Services, Dr. Eric Keroack, said "people who have misused their sexual faculty and become bonded to multiple persons will diminish the power of oxytocin to maintain a permanent bond with an individual."[11] Dr. Keroack's main concern was preventing promiscuity in women, which he blamed for the high rates of divorce and unhappy marriages, suggesting that these problems emerged from an acquired tolerance or insensitivity to the effects of oxytocin.

Dopamine and serotonin are two other important neurochemicals, intensely involved in both cognitive and emotional brain activity. Disturbances in these two chemicals are involved in the development of depression, and other neurological disorders. Studies using MRI images of individuals looking at pictures of their new loves show that the brain pumps out more dopamine when the individual looks at images of the person with whom they've recently fallen in love. High levels of dopamine are also often associated with higher levels of norepinephrine. Norepinephrine is a chemical pretty close to what we call adrenaline, contributing to those high levels of energy and excitement, when we first fall in love.

Interestingly, the levels of serotonin work in the opposite direction—when a person is newly in love, their serotonin levels drop, leading an individual to be more preoccupied with their new love, and more impulsive and reckless in their behavior, particularly when it comes to being with their new lover. Most of the current antidepressant drugs, known as selective serotonin reuptake inhibitors (SSRIs), like Prozac, have strong antilibido side effects. In women, they often decrease sexual arousal and response, and can even lead to migraine responses to orgasm. In men, they have a pronounced effect on the ability to achieve an erection, as well as decreasing one's interest in sex. These drugs increase the amount of serotonin in a person's brain. When a person has more dopamine in their brain (as happens when they are newly falling in love or lust), they are more sexual, more emotionally reactive, more impulsive, and perhaps, more stimulating to both current and new sexual partners.

But, the brain (and our sexual organs) would likely burn out if the levels of PEA, oxytocin, and dopamine stayed at those high levels. Somewhere between six months and two years after a romantic relationship begins, the brain neurochemistry starts to change. Dopamine starts to decrease, and serotonin increases. This is when, after the first heady weeks and months of an intense relationship, we start to think again (and sometimes realize that we've leapt headlong into a pretty crazy relationship). Another neurochemical, vasopressin, becomes more prevalent in the brain in the days and weeks following sexual intimacy, and seems to be more related to attachment, nurturing, cuddling, and monogamy. Vasopressin starts to replace oxytocin, and suppresses the high levels of dopamine and norepinephrine. (Very high levels of vasopressin can also interfere in the production of norepinephrine and dopamine—thus, the decrease in lusty sex drive, as attachment and bonding increases.)

When vasopressin is increased in prairie voles, they are more likely to persist in monogamous mating, even when that mating produces no offspring, and are far less promiscuous. Vasopressin may increase the likelihood that males and females will bond, in order to safely gestate, birth, nurture, and rear offspring. Males with more vasopressin are less likely to chase off after other females. In humans, vasopressin is also present during lactation, as a mother breast-feeds, and may stimulate the "bonding" that happens for the mother, as she feeds her child.

In males, higher levels of testosterone predict libido and sex drive (and increased domestic violence and divorce). When a father holds or interacts with his infant child, testosterone levels decrease immediately. This might well serve to prevent or reduce infanticide, but might also contribute to the decreased sexual activity reported by many couples postpartum.

In males, levels of vasopressin increase dramatically after mating. They don't increase comparably in females after sexual intercourse (instead, female production of oxytocin increases—I wonder if this root difference has anything to do with Galen's comment that only women are not "sad" after sex), suggesting that there may be more evolutionary need to chemically stimulate a mating, pair-bonding behavior in males following mating than females. Research published in 2008 from Stockholm reported that the presence of certain genes related to vasopressin production in males predicted the marital satisfaction ratings of those males offered by their wives. In other words, males whose genes interfered in the production of effective levels of vasopressin tended to have marriages that were less positive and healthy, and had wives who were generally less satisfied with their husband's role in their marriage.

Many couples describe how their interests in sexual relationships outside their marriage begin as the "sexual energy" and excitement in their marriage has begun to decline. Might it be that these individuals are somehow seeking increased release of that heady neurochemical cocktail they felt when they first fell in love? Some writers and researchers suggest that when couples do exciting, dangerous, and thrilling activities together, their brain chemistries resemble those early days of falling in love, with high levels of adrenaline, and the oxytocin associated with engaging in risky, impulsive behaviors. Many swinging, hotwifing, and nonmonogamous couples report that after sexual relationships with others, they often return home and "relive the experience," having renewed sexual excitement with each other. In the 1970s, both *Cosmopolitan* and *Playboy* recommended to readers that extramarital affairs could put the "spark" back in their marriage. Might it be that that spark is comprised of the chemicals released in lust? Oxytocin, norepinephrine, and dopamine? I'd love to see studies of the neurochemistry of nonmonogamous couples, investigating the levels of oxytocin before, during, and after extramarital sex. And, in those couples where the extramarital sex is open and negotiated, is vasopressin more present in their brains when they "cuddle" and renew their relationship with each other after having sex with others?

Research with animals and humans shows that male sexual drive, frequency of intercourse, and attention to the female goes up as the presence of other males around the female increases. As with the increased production of sperm when a male's mate is away from him, or having sex with other males, so too does the male's interest in having sex with the female increase. Sexual interest and libido are mediated in the body by the influence of hormones and neurochemicals. Wife sharing and the cuckold lifestyle may serve an adaptive function for the couple by increasing and maintaining the husband's virility and sexual interest in his wife, along with the level of attention he pays to his wife.

It may not be just the neurochemicals, but there may be structural influences in the brain that support and encourage female promiscuity. Some women with epilepsy have suffered lesions, or damage, to a part of their temporal lobe, damage that has sometimes led to severe promiscuity. Another type of brain dysfunction, Klüver-Bucy syndrome, involves damage to another part of the brain, the amygdala, a part of the brain involved in emotional functioning. This sometimes results from stroke, or sometimes after brain surgery. Klüver-Bucy syndrome sometimes results in a tremendous increase in lust and hypersexual behaviors that are often random and difficult to control. Research has suggested that the amygdala also plays a role in male voyeurism. When research participants are shown explicit sexual imagery, the male amygdala responds with far more neurochemical activity than it does in females. So, males appear to be biologically predisposed to respond more with greater neurological excitement to voyeuristic and visual sexual imagery. Watching someone engage in sexual activity may be, by nature, more innately rewarding for males.

The fertile fluids of the genitals, semen, and female prostatic fluids represent the current status of the "arms race" between male and female sexual development, a race centered around the effects of cuckoldry. The heady brew of the effects of these fluids, involved as they are with feelings of sexual pleasure and arousal, are certainly involved in the physiological and psychological experiences of these couples, as their behaviors trigger biological responses within their bodies that heighten their sexual arousal and enhance the sexual adventures they pursue within, and without, their marriages. Some people appear to have dispositions that lead them to seek novelty in sexual and intimate interactions, more so than others. These individuals, due perhaps to a heightened sensitivity to oxytocin, or perhaps a decreased effect or presence of vasopressin, or some as yet unknown physiological function, are physiologically disinclined towards monogamy. They may then pursue covert extra-relationship sexual activity, or they may engage their partner in discussion of one of the various forms of negotiated nonmonogamy, such as swinging, open marriages, polyamory, or hotwifing.

Couples describe the decline of sexuality within their marriages, and watching their sex lives become "nonexistent." One husband reflected that he only began to see his wife as a sexual person again when he began to entertain the fantasies of her being with other men. He saw her as a friend and companion, but found that fantasizing about her being sexual with other men kept him "focused" on her as a sexual being, despite his wife having no idea as to the origin of his renewed sexual interest.[12] Similarly, other couples confirm that maintaining the excitement that exists early in relationships is impossible. Recovering the "butterfly in stomach" feeling of early love and sex with a new lover is a valuable, often intentional, side effect of engaging in swinging and nonmonogamous sex. One husband shared that seeing his wife in sexual bliss is the greatest reward for him, and that both he and his wife experience tremendous satisfaction from the encounters. In his words, "I would trade all my own sexual freedom for the intense satisfaction of watching my wife meet, flirt, seduce, and have crazy, wild, frantic screaming orgasms with other men."[13]

MADONNA
OR WHORE?

*While I can't prove it, I think that middle-class American hus-
bands now, more than ever before in American history, can live
with the knowledge that their wives were not virgins when they
married—and that their wives have had, or are having, an extramarital affair. I'm not saying that these husbands are not
bothered by this. . . . I'm only suggesting that the contemporary
husband, unlike his father and grandfather before him, is not so
shocked or shattered by such news, is more likely to accept women
as sexual beings, and only in extreme cases will he retaliate with
violence against his unfaithful wife or male rival.*

Gay Talese, *Thy Neighbor's Wife*[1]

In his work *Contributions to the Psychology of Love*, Sigmund Freud described the concept of the Madonna–whore complex, and the role it
had in male infidelity. Freud suggested that some men resolved the Oedipal conflict, the struggle over sharing their mother with their father, by
developing an image of their mother as a saint-like figure, sexless, altruistic, and pure. As that male child developed sexual feelings, they drew
defining lines between women who were "for" sex, and those who were
not. A woman with whom one could enjoy sex, and who could herself
enjoy sex, was quite different from the woman who could raise one's children. Thus, once a man had children with his wife, he now began to view
his wife in the same terms that he viewed his mother, seeing her as a

Madonna, and unavailable to him sexually. So, this man might then pursue sexual encounters with other women, who were free in his mind to be a whore, to enjoy and embrace sexuality, with no conflict. Sex is "dirty," and reserved for "dirty" women.

Men want their wives to be a lady in the drawing room, impressing their friends; a maid in the kitchen, cooking their food; and a whore in the bedroom, with whom the men can enjoy unfettered and unrestrained sexuality. In Brazil, they want a saint in the family room, and a piranha in the bed. A psychodynamic view of the Madonna–whore complex suggests that men seek out women whose characteristics resemble their mother. However, in the bedroom, the resemblance to their mother interferes in their sexual arousal. So, in order to get aroused, the husband either seeks sexual gratification with other (dirty) women, or encourages his wife to act "like a whore" in the bedroom. Because his or her mother would not, of course, ever act in such a way, the male is then able to short-circuit this conflict, see his wife as someone different from his mother, and achieve sexual arousal. Further, by seeing his wife as a sexual object, the man acknowledges internally that his wife might be attractive to other men, and thus, he must compete for her attention, just as he competed with his father for his mother's attention.

Husbands of some wives have gone further, allowing their wife to carry the "whore" image outside the bedroom, or invited other men into the bedroom to share their wife's sexuality, taking that "whore" concept to its ultimate limit. One Tennessee couple with whom I corresponded embraced this concept so fully after the husband shared his wife with another man on their honeymoon that the wife now works a week or two a month at a Nevada brothel. In 2006, a fifty-eight-year-old German housewife took a job in a brothel, saying: "I like sex, I like it a lot, but my husband Ginther has no appetite for sex anymore and does it about once a year." Her husband "Ginther's not thrilled about it, but I can't hem myself in just because he's not up for it and we're actually getting on better now."[2]

In Uri Wernik's research, he suggests that this dichotomy is evident in about 35 percent of the letters and fantasies he analyzed. By watching their wives lose their sexual inhibitions, he hypothesizes that these men may have become increasingly able to connect with their wives in a sexual way. Though Wernik does not suggest this, I wonder if the finding that these men desired to free their wives of sexual restraint had more to do with freeing the husbands' ability to view their wives in a sexual manner, and less about the wife's actual sexual capacity or behavior.

Evolutionary researcher David Buss has partnered with David Schmitt to study the characteristics of both men and women who "poach" on the relationships of others, seeking out sexual relationships with individuals already in relationships. In cultures that are more egalitarian, women and men engage in "mate-poaching" almost equally, though in cultures where women have less independence and fewer protections, this practice is almost exclusively reserved to men. According to their research, in North America, 62 percent of men and 40 percent of women (another study found that 53 percent of women admit to attempted poaching) have tried to entice a person in a monogamous relationship, into a sexual relationship with them. Half of all men, and a third of women report that they have accepted such invitations from poachers.

Poachers and poachees share some common characteristics, in that they both tend to be open to new experiences and stimulated by novelty, open about talking about sexuality, and sexually attractive. The poachers did not tend to be nice people. Schmitt described both male and female poachers as "disagreeable, untrusting, immodest, harsh-minded, mean, unreliable, adulterous and highly focused on sex."[3] Men and women who were in committed relationships but were willing to be "poached" (sorry, I just keep thinking of a saucepan, poaching eggs—"This is your relationship on extramarital sex") were also not the nicest people. Marius, the male lover in Howard Jacobson's book, is a prototypical mate poacher. They tended to have high levels of self-esteem, but were rated as untrustworthy, immodest, deceptive, and rather selfish. Both poachers and poachees used a similar strategy at times, destabilizing the poached relationship by inviting the poacher to "meddle" in the relationship. When the poacher, under the guise of trying to help a troubled relationship, stirred up more problems, the poacher was then able to swoop in and comfort the target of their affections.

I suspect that this research sheds some light on a surprising report made by many of the nonmonogamous couples I interviewed. Many couples told me that it was a lot harder for them to find an appealing man who would have sex with the wife when the husband was consenting. "You'd think most men would jump at the chance to have no-strings attached sex with my wife!" I suggest that the men who were willing to have sex with the wives, and were found by these couples, might have resembled these poachers. Particularly when ovulating, women find most attractive those confident men who are also somewhat condescending to other men. So, there may be a potential conflict between the desires of the wife to find an outside male lover that meets her unconscious desires for genetic success, and her husband's desires for a man with whom he feels he can safely share his wife. The men they find might tend to be the somewhat disagreeable, mean, sexually focused, and generally untrustworthy men who are generally happy to seduce another man's wife, though usually without the husband's consent or awareness.

In addition, despite the availability of "no strings attached" sex with another man's wife, more men are likely to decline than one might initially think. Though men tend to be far more interested in short-term sexual encounters than women, research suggests that men are least likely to choose women for such encounters, when the woman's characteristics are such that there is a greater likelihood of sperm competition. In other words, even when looking for an no-strings-attached quickie, men unconsciously prefer women where their sperm has a greater chance of entering an "empty playing field." When the woman is obviously married or partnered, there is a greater chance that the man's sperm will hit the field, as it were, and have to compete with the "home team." Other studies have shown that single men are less likely to find married women sexually attractive.

Several couples suggested to me that outside men have been "scared off" when the couple was honest about their relationship and intentions. They said that many men simply can't believe a man would share his wife, and can't understand a situation they think might be potentially dangerous. More men are willing to cheat with a wife, than are willing to participate with a voluntary sharing or cuckolding arrangement.

As one couple told me, more important issues may involve the character of the other man: "You have to be able to trust this other man. You're inviting him into your home, your life, and your wife's bed. He has to be the kind of person you can have dinner with." In addition, I suspect that these men, and other men who wouldn't fit the characteristics of a poacher, might be instinctively assuming that these wives fit the profile of a "poacher," in being deceptive and selfish. The intelligent, respectful, and trustworthy man that many of these couples say they are seeking might be assuming that a wife who would engage in such behaviors is like other wives who "cheat" on their husbands. These men, not fitting any of the characteristics of the typical poacher, might be unlikely to be attracted to such women, and thus reject the wife or couple's overtures. However, in this different kind of relationship, where extramarital sex and promiscuity are not secret, but an accepted part of the relationship, I'm not so sure these old rules apply. These relationships, and the wives in particular, appear to be based on very high degrees of trust and communication, with remarkably little deception.

Steve Gangestad, an evolutionary psychologist and former professor of mine, proposes a mating strategy he sometimes calls "dad vs. cad." He argues that males blessed with high degrees of bilateral symmetry, a measure of the degree to which one side of the face most closely matches the other side, may have greater ability to implement a selfish reproductive strategy. Bilateral symmetry, which is very predictive of the degree to which women find a given male attractive, predicts male number of sexual partners, infidelity, and even the time it takes for a man to get a woman into bed. Men with high degrees of bilateral symmetry may choose to act out a "cad" strategy, bouncing from woman to woman, lying to her to procure sex.

Men with lower levels of bilateral symmetry may instead be limited to the "dad" strategy, mating with a woman, and staying with her, providing for her and their child, in order to secure reproductive success for his genes. Meanwhile, the woman is often sneakily involved in sexual encounters outside of the relationship with those "cads." Thus, in evolutionary history, the wife-sharing lifestyle represents an ideal strategy for a woman, but not her husband or mate. She gets to "sample" lots of virile, handsome, strong males who wouldn't make good husbands, while still having her "good" husband at home to raise her kids. In the words of evolutionary researcher D. C. Geary, "women must balance the costs of reduced paternal investment or male retaliation against the benefits of cuckoldry; that is, having their children sired by a more fit man while having their social partner assist in the rearing of those children."

One husband shared with me that it was fascinating to have his wife be with another man, who was more successful than he, the husband, was. The couple had done this for long enough that the husband did not struggle with envy or jealousy, but instead found it fascinating to be proud of his wife for having such a successful lover. Further, the husband acknowledged that he achieved a sense of "one-upmanship" as his wife left this successful man to return to him, making him the "alpha," and the better man, no matter how powerful or successful or arrogant the other lover was.[4]

In the reproductive behaviors of redback spiders, the male sacrifices himself, devoured alive by the female, *while* the male copulates with her. The males that can last longest, and sacrifice themselves, pass on more sperm to the female, and are more likely to have their genes carried on by another generation. Those male redback spiders that live to mate another day and don't die in the arms of their mate? They pass on fewer sperm to the female, and are thus less likely to reproduce.

Is the submissive male in these hotwife couples exerting a sacrificial reproductive strategy? Are these women, for instance, more attractive than the male is powerful or dominant, such that in normal situations, this male could not hope to mate with this woman? Could the husband here be sacrificing monogamy, to the hope that by putting his sperm in the mix, he has a better chance of reproducing with this woman, and mixing his genes with hers? In other words, is this a version of "marrying-up," whereby a person accepts some flaw of their partner, in order to "marry-up" a level with a mate who is more wealthy, powerful, or attractive than they?

In British studies, females who are unfaithful to their husbands most often choose external mates who are more successful, and of higher status, than their husbands. Women very rarely choose extramarital mates among men of lower class than their husbands (in contrast to the standard jokes about the pool man).

British evolutionary scientist Robin Baker has described this possibility, suggesting that in birds, females almost always seem to give their primary mate at least a chance to sire children with her. In humans, a similar pattern emerges, in that in families with multiple children, the second child is most likely to be biologically related to the father. The first child and especially the last child are least likely to have been fathered by the mother's husband.

A similar, but related argument might explain why most studies have shown that swingers tend to be older, and already have children. It might be that both women and men find swinging "safer" when they have already had children together. For the male, he is already assured of his own reproduction. For the female, she may be assured of her husband's continued "paternal support," even if she were to become impregnated by another man.

Swinging, hotwifing, polyamory, and other forms of nonmonogamous relationships, may offer individuals the ability to act out or live the "perks" of extreme social/economic success. They can choose to claim the monogamy rule exemption that has been "awarded" to kings, queens, presidents, rulers, chief executive officers, and millionaires throughout history. By acting temporarily like a sultan with a harem, or a "queen bee" with a hive full of male subjects, the individual may be unconsciously seeking the internal, and possibly external, esteem that comes with these levels of social success and power. As such, they can be "pretenders to the throne of reproductive dominance," as phrased by Joann Rodgers, author of *Sex: A Natural History*.[5]

Iris Brent, housewife from Chicago, left her husband and moved to California to embrace the free love movement, and published her autobiography, *Swinger's Diary*, in 1973, where, after being the center of an interracial orgy with five black men, she wrote that:

> As their semen spurted out over my body, and Roger's began to drain out of my vagina, I felt drowned in sex. . . . I felt like a princess who had just been anointed queen—like the center of the universe, warm, happy, and oh so very satisfied."[6]

Online, one can spend around five hundred dollars to purchase the "Queening Chair," a well-designed, handmade chair that is designed to allow a woman to sit up regally, and comfortably, while she receives cunnilingus (or analingus, the site notes) from a lover.[7] The site is maintained and owned by a woman, who proudly points out that each piece is personally "tested" by herself and her cuckold lover. Designed with the cuckolding couple in mind, the chair is intended to provide a comfortable sexual aid, but also, to support the power differential held by a "cuckoldress" over her lover.

In *The Lifestyle*, by Steven Gould, Patti Johnson, a swinger and organizer of swinging social events, is quoted as saying, "a woman gets to be treated like a queen, and a guy gets to feel he's married to a queen, with all the guys wanting what he's got."[8] Gould also cites a 1970s sex researcher, Dr. Gilbert Bartell, who argued that "swinging was the appropriation by the middle class of what the media constantly advertised as the chief privilege of celebrity: the license to indulge in royal revelry, which was refused to commoners. The people the media sold the dream to *were* the bourgeoisie, and the bourgeoisie *were* the swingers."[9] In pursuing swinging sexual activity, the middle class were mimicking the lifestyles of the modern American royalty, the Hollywood star.

In his research with the writers of wife-sharing letters, Israeli psychologist Uri Werik found that many men were able to find a measure of peace in the knowledge that they can "see himself as a winner in a competition with other males, as he is the one to stay home after the other ones are gone." Several men with whom I corresponded shared similar feelings, that they felt powerful and aroused, watching other men desire their wives, knowing that in the end, she "chose" them.

Evolutionary researcher Aaron Goetz has found that men partnered with women who are likely to be sexually unfaithful often use "sexual inducements" as a means to maintain and retain their partner's fidelity. These sexual inducements include most often, giving in to their partner's sexual requests, and performing "sexual favors to keep her around." Goetz suggests that these husbands apply these methods as a "corrective tactic," in order to create opportunities where the husbands' sperm might enter into "competition" with any sperm from other men present in their partners' body.[10] In other words, Goetz suggests that these men may enter into a Hobbsian bargain, where they accept their wife might be sexually unfaithful, but attempt to increase the chances that at least they will get to have sex with their wife too, and thereby increase the opportunity their sperm will have to get on the field and defend their territory, as it were.

In yet another study with that lusty little critter, the prairie vole, researchers at Emory University in Atlanta found that by transferring a single gene into the part of the brain that governs pleasure, they were able to transform a previously nonmonogamous male into the loyal, stay-at-home vole husband that every female vole wants. While the researchers avoided the idea of gene therapy for straying spouses, they did suggest that their research may help inform therapy with conditions such as autism, personality disorders, and attachment disorders, where people have problems developing a bond with others.

Provocative studies have supported the genetic heritability of non-monogamous behaviors, or at least, infidelity. Identical twins are 40 percent likely to report having engaged in extramarital sex if their identical sibling has also engaged in sex outside their relationship. Some people, by the complex, multidetermined course of nature and nurture, with the commingled influences of brain structures and neurochemicals, the influences of genes and evolutionarily determined strategies, along with life experiences, traumas, successes, and role models, appear disposed against lifelong monogamy. For those individuals, different paths can be chosen. The first fork in the road is whether or not their sexual activity will be secret from their partner. If it is secret, there is a long, well-trodden path before them, the road mapped out before them by countless men and women. The other path is far less trodden, and involves many forks within it. If they approach their partner or spouse, at the beginning of their relationship or any point within, they begin to steer towards one the options within negotiated non-monogamy. Along this path, trodden by agreement of both partners, they have choices about what kinds of relationships and encounters they may have. Will they involve sexual encounters only, or will they be allowed or encouraged to develop into the aspects of emotional intimacy? Who will their partners be, and where will they find them? Will both partners be involved in these outside relationships, together or apart, or is this a road that only one will truly walk, while the other strides along beside the road, supporting and enjoying their partner's journey?

Any complex human behavior is invariably multiply determined, with many different causes, and many different effects. Attempts to reduce the sexual practices of nonmonogamous wives with consenting, even encouraging husbands to a single, simple answer are bound to be wrong far more often than they are right. Calling this behavior an outgrowth of voyeurism, or exhibitionism, or even masochism, is only likely to explain a small percentage of the cases, and also likely to answer only a very few of the questions that it will raise.

Contrary to the social belief that cuckoldry is rare, and that accepted sexual infidelity by wives is even rarer, there is a long, long history of husbands who actively and passively allow their wives to take other lovers. Though many of the recorded historical incidents of this occurred in artistic, literati, and intelligentsia communities, there are records that suggest this lifestyle and sexual practice may have been present throughout social levels and classes. It may be that the taboo associated with these behaviors prevented many individuals and couples from pursuing it, or openly acknowledging it if they did. The current apparent prevalence of this lifestyle may reflect a change in the social prohibitions, or it might simply reflect an increased freedom of expression of these behaviors, through the anonymous, democratic, and "free" forum of the Internet.

The practice of wife sharing, hotwifing, or cuckoldry is not inherently pathological or destructive. Indeed, couples who are able to pursue this lifestyle successfully for long periods of time tend to have extremely healthy relationships, and extraordinary patterns of communication within their marriage. While this lifestyle can and does sometimes stem from emotional or relationship disturbance, it may just as often be neutral, or even serve an adaptive function, helping individuals and couples to overcome things such as fear, issues of power and control, the need for freedom and independence, and the need to give up power and the burden of meeting social expectations.

Wives who pursue this lifestyle find themselves confronting not only the complex expectations of monogamy and marriage, but also the millennia of social expectations and directions toward women. In some surprising ways, this lifestyle includes complex, powerful messages of feminism and female empowerment, beyond mere sexuality. Women in our culture are pressured to live a duality, to be nice and, sometimes, to be not nice. To be sexy, but not too sexy. Some of the wives who embrace a version of wife sharing, have found a power in it, a power to reject what society says they must be, and to define for themselves, who and what they choose to be.

Marriage and family therapist Beverly Engel recently published *The Nice Girl Syndrome*, describing the prevalence of pressure upon women to be "nice." By Engel's definition, being nice usually means worrying about others' needs; sacrificing for others instead of yourself; letting other people walk all over you; and hiding or suppressing anger for fear of being labeled, ostracized, blamed, or rejected. Engel argues that being nice, as women are taught from childhood, has been protective in the past, protecting women from men, and reducing conflict with other women. Like the arguments made by Baumeister and Twenge, being nice allowed women to cooperate without fighting over men. But, in today's society, being nice is far less protective than it once was. Some women, like Kay, Bobby, and other women whose stories are told here, have found that pursuing their own sexual fulfillment, without regard for the primary needs of their husbands, has led to an independence, a freedom from the need to be nice, the need to constantly seek and maintain approval, and to ruffle no feathers. And, as Engel argues, sometimes being independent and powerful also involves being selfish, being bad, and accepting all sides of oneself, both good and bad.

There is a powerful independence in many of these women, an independence that, by many of their accounts, was absent or hidden before their husbands began to encourage them to seek sexual fulfillment outside their marriage. As these women embrace other men, initially to fulfill their husband's fantasy, something is freed within them. Sexuality, is in many ways, a symbol. It is a symbol of love, relationship, selfishness, self-worth, and value to others. Sexuality incorporates, and represents, much of what makes us human, and how we live our lives. It includes much of what is good in people, but doesn't exclude that dark side, our social issues with sexism, racism, and violence. As these women have rejected those powerful early messages, that "nice" girls don't like sex, or at least not too much, and certainly not sex outside their marriage, these women have, in some ways, opened doors that allow them to explore many other aspects of themselves, only tangentially connected to sexuality.

Female sexuality has, at its core, a receptive, reactive nature. Males, with less sexual capacity than females, show far greater interest in the pursuit and initiation of sex than do women. Some couples described to me that the female sexual engine is harder to get turned on, but that once it is revved-up, the horsepower far outstripped that of the male engine. In a nice match, males are more oriented towards giving sexual pleasure than are females. While my wife points out that this portrays men as more sexually altruistic than they are, I think that this characteristic is not based upon altruism, but on the internal needs fulfilled when a man gives pleasure to a woman. His esteem and "manliness" are enhanced; he may feel less fear that she will need to seek sexual fulfillment away from him; his satisfaction may even relate to an evolutionary connection between the female orgasm and fertilization. Husbands of many of these wives enhance their satisfaction, through vicarious participation in their wife's sexual fulfillment. These husbands, in part, are able, by proxy of their wife, to reach beyond the limits of male sexual capacity, to experience the far greater range of sexual fulfillment available to women.

Wives and their husbands live in a modern world where female sexuality is a complex, multifaceted construct that varies for each woman. Female sexuality, while it may still engender fear and intimidation, is now a celebrated and cherished part of many couples' physical and emotional relationships.

There are many reasons and causes for these couples' pursuit of this lifestyle. One common effect persists across these couples, that of heightened sexual pleasure within their own relationship. They have stumbled, unconsciously, upon the use of complex methods to enhance and maintain high levels of sexual excitement in their marriage. Without knowing the means, only the cause and the effect, these couples have developed a sophisticated dance that uses biological and psychological methods to increase the husband's desire for his wife, and his sexual performance, and for the wife to enhance and pursue the depths of her own sexual capacity. They have unconsciously hit upon a script that uses neurochemical triggers, psychological responses such as jealousy, biological responses such as increased sperm production, and other complex interplays between the different parts of our bodies and minds. This script works from the principles and tools that are in our genes and bodies, our psyches and our hearts, all designed and intended to increase the chances that we will mate, fall in love, have children, raise them together, and die together one day. But, these couples have found ways to turn these tools, these tricks of our bodies and minds, completely upon their heads. This lifestyle offers a real-life laboratory, in which one can observe the influence and effects of the many, many biological, social, relational, and cognitive mechanisms that are interwoven within the fabric of sexuality within a marriage.

As I worked on this book, I encountered various reactions, from friends and colleagues. Most reacted with feelings and thoughts similar to my initial responses, concerned that these couples were driven by mental health problems, marital conflict, or male desire to escape sexual monogamy. Others were surprised and intrigued as I described some of my more interesting findings and interviews. My father's response was one of the more interesting, as he said, "You're writing about what? Are you crazy? You can't go writing about this. Every husband in the world will want to chop your head off, because all their wives are going to want this too!" There is a strong secretiveness to this behavior, and a sense that society doesn't want to acknowledge that this exists. And yet, despite this long, often bloody history, there are, and always have been, husbands who encouraged their wives to have sex with other men. This work explores the history of cuckoldry, and describes couples, past and present, that have not only accepted, but celebrated, the wives' sexual encounters with other men. Currently, many couples and individuals are using the Internet to explore, document, and discuss their sexual adventures. Their practices open the doors to a long-held secret of marital sexuality.

One might suggest that these couples are playing with fire, a hot, green fire, whose flames are jealousy, envy, and possessiveness. Indeed, I think many, if not most, people would be unable to play with these flames as successfully and burn-free as some of these couples manage. But, these couples may be like the people who walk across hot coals, and find that so long as they keep moving, the coals do not transmit enough heat to burn them. Pursuit of sexuality outside a marriage, through cuckoldry or hotwifing, is not inherently unhealthy. These couples can be successful, so long as they keep moving, keep communicating, maintain a healthy relationship, and acknowledge those flames of jealousy and envy as cues and signals, not as obstacles. There is nothing different in this from any other relationship. The things these couples do to remain healthy are the same things any couple should do. Health in relationships is determined not by what a couple does together, but how they communicate with each other, how they treat each other, and how they work together to maintain a functioning, mutually beneficial relationship. Communication, freedom, support, and mutual regard are the key components to any healthy relationship, regardless of sexual behaviors.

ENDNOTES

CHAPTER ONE

1. Todd Shackelford and Aaron Goetz, "Predicting Violence against Women from Men's Mate-retention Behaviors," in *Female Infidelity and Paternal Uncertainty*, ed. Platek and Shackelford (New York: Cambridge University Press, 2006), 58–81.

2. Richard von Krafft-Ebing, *Psychopathia Sexualis, with Especial Reference to Contrary Sexual Instinct: A Medico-legal Study.* Translated by Charles Gilbert Chaddock. 1894. http://books.google.com/books?id=azotAAAAYAAJ andprintsec=frontcoveranddq=Psychopathia+sexualis:+Contrary+sexual +instincts.+A+medico-legal+study.#PPR1,M1.

3. "Races: What We Call Cornuto," http://www.time.com/time/magazine/article/0,9171,760456,00.html.

4. http://www.urbandictionary.com/define.php?term=WITTOL.

5. Claudia Fonseca, "Philanderers, Cuckolds, and Wily Women," *Men and Masculinities* 3, no. 3 (2001): 261–277.

6. Richard Zacks, *History Laid Bare: Love, Sex, and Perversity from the Ancient Romans to Warren G. Harding* (New York: HarperCollins, 1994), 169.

7. Zacks, *History Laid Bare*, 169.

8. G. R. Quaife, *Wanton Wenches and Wayward Wives: Peasants and Illicit Sex in Early Seventeenth Century England* (New Brunswick, N.J.: Rutgers University Press, 1979), 157.

9. Quaife, *Wanton Wenches and Wayward Wives*, 157.

10. Quaife, *Wanton Wenches and Wayward Wives*, 157.

11. Quaife, *Wanton Wenches and Wayward Wives*, 157.

12. Quaife, *Wanton Wenches and Wayward Wives*, 157.

13. Quaife, *Wanton Wenches and Wayward Wives*, 151.

14. Quaife, *Wanton Wenches and Wayward Wives*, 153.

15. Judith Warner, "Horned and Scorned," *New York Times*, September 13, 2007.

16. Ellis O'Hanlon, "Sarkozy's Critics Fail to See He Just Needs a Life," http://www.independent.ie/opinion/analysis/sarkozys-criticis-fail-to-see-he-just-needs-a-life-1264936.html (accessed March 29, 2009).

CHAPTER TWO

1. Ria Lemaire quoted by Marilyn Yalom, *A History of the Wife* (New York: HarperCollins, 2001), 69.

2. T. Lewin, "In Genetic Testing for Paternity, Law Often Lags Behind Science," *New York Times*, March 11, 2001.

CHAPTER THREE

1. Havelock Ellis, *Little Essays of Love and Virtue*, http://www.gutenberg.org/ebooks/15687 (2005, accessed March 21, 2009).

2. http://en.wikipedia.org/wiki/Tiresias (accessed March 21, 2009).

3. Heinrich Kramer and James Sprenger, *Malleus Maleficarum*, http://www.malleusmaleficarum.org/ (accessed March 21, 2009).

4. Mark Twain, *Letters From the Earth*, http://www.sacred-texts.com/aor/twain/letearth.htm (accessed March 23, 2009).

5. www.allgreatquotes.com/mae_west_quotes4.shtml (accessed March 19, 2009).

6. capt_spongefoot, http://ourhotwives.org/forum/viewtopic.php?f=6&t=5176&p=71285&hilit=bite+marks#p712851 (accessed January 16, 2008).

7. L. Barber, "Girls Hated Sex. So I Was Told," *The Observer*, December 7, 2008.

8. Joe Sonka, "Slutty Girls Seducing Stupid Boys: Yet Another Absurd, Sexist Fallacy of Abstinence-Only Education," AlterNet.org, March 10, 2009, http://www.alternet.org/sex/130962/ (accessed March 18, 2009).

9. Michele Weiner-Davis, *The Sex-Starved Wife* (New York: Simon & Schuster, 2008), 165.

10. Roy Baumeister and Jean Twenge, "Cultural Suppression of Female Sexuality," *Review of General Psychology* 6, no. 2 (2002): 166–203, 172.

11. Havelock Ellis, *Studies in the Psychology of Sex*, vol. 3, http://manybooks.net/titles/ellishav13611361213612-8.html (accessed March 1, 2009), 319.

12. Marty Klein, *America's War on Sex, The Attack on Law, Lust and Liberty* (Westport, Conn.: Praeger Publishers, 2008), 89.

13. Carol Groneman, *Nymphomania, A History* (New York: W. W. Norton, 2000), 71.

14. James H. Jones, *Alfred C. Kinsey, A Public/Private Life* (New York: W. W. Norton, 1997), 693.

15. C. Panati, *Sexy Origins and Intimate Things* (New York, Penguin Books, 1998), 31.

16. Daniel Bergner, "What Do Women Want?" *New York Times Magazine*, January 22, 2009.

17. Gay Talese, *Thy Neighbor's Wife* (New York: Dell, 1980), 404.

18. Dalma Heyn, *The Erotic Silence of the American Wife* (New York: Turtle Bay Books, 1992), 46.

19. A. Levin, "Infidelity: Being Unfaithful Keeps Me Happy," *Telegraph*, January 24, 2008.

20. matt2, http://ourhotwives.org/forum/viewtopic.php?f=5&t=5344&p=72105&hilit=abundant+sex+appeal#p72105 (accessed November 25, 2008).

21. diane, http://ourhotwives.org/forum/viewtopic.php?f=5&t=113&p=22228&hilit=right+of+refusal#p22228 (accessed September 20, 2007).

22. Aaron Goetz and Todd Shackelford, "Sperm Competition and Its Evolutionary Consequences in Humans," in *Female Infidelity and Paternal Uncertainty,* ed. Platek and Shackelford (New York: Cambridge University Press, 2006), 111.

INTERLUDE 3

1. princess, http://ourhotwives.org/forum/viewtopic.php?f=5&t=5076&p=70408&hilit=princess+balance+of+power#p70408 (accessed November 7, 2008).

CHAPTER 4

1. http://www.brainyquote.com/quotes/keywords/monogamy.html (accessed September 25, 2008).

2. K. Freeman, "Science Watch: Make Room for Daddies," *New York Times*, March 10, 1998.

3. Martin Luther, "*A Prelude by Martin Luther on the Babylonian Captivity of the Church*," Project Wittenberg Online Electronic Study Edition, http://www.ctsfw.edu/etext/luther/babylonian/babylonian.htm (accessed March 1, 2009).

4. mdcucked, http://ourhotwives.org (accessed January 19, 2009).

5. Terry Gould, *The Lifestyle, A Look at the Erotic Rites of Swingers* (Buffalo, N.Y.: Firefly, 2000), 174.

6. Linda Wolfe, *Playing Around: Women and Extramarital Sex* (New York: William Morrow and Company, 1975), 216.

7. Wolfe, *Playing Around*, 216.

8. Wolfe, *Playing Around*, 217.

9. Wolfe, *Playing Around*, 220–221.

10. Wolfe, *Playing Around*, 221.

11. Robert Heinlein, *Stranger in a Strange Land* (New York: Putnam, 1961), 450.

12. CTSubOralHub, http://ourhotwives.org/forum/viewtopic.php?f=6&t=3182&p=43183&hilit=vanilla+prejudiced#p43183 (accessed February 29, 2008).

13. http://en.wikipedia.org/wiki/Hotwife (accessed March 20, 2009).

14. http://en.wikipedia.org/wiki/Hotwife (accessed March 20, 2009).

15. Badhubby2, http://bb4.redclouds.com//messages/15288957/15288957.html?1097145655 (accessed September 14, 2008).

INTERLUDE 4

1. Flaguy, e-mail message to author, September 14, 2008.

CHAPTER 5

1. Simone de Beauvoir, *The Second Sex*, trans. H. M. Parshley (1952; reprint, New York: Vintage, 1989), 396.

2. Burgo Partridge, *A History of Orgies* (1958; reprint, London: Sevenoaks, 2005).

3. http://www.goups.dcs.st-and.ac.uk/~history/Biographies/chatelet.htm (accessed October 4, 2008).

4. Zacks, *History Laid Bare*, 381.

5. www.lkwdpl.org/wihohio/wood-vic.htm (accessed November 8, 2008).

6. Marguerite, Countess of Blessington, 1789–1849, *A Journal of Conversations with Lord Byron with a sketch of the life of the author*, http://www
.archive.org/stream/journalofconvers00blesuoft/journalofconvers00
blesuoft_djvu.txt (accessed March 23, 2009).

7. Quoted in Wolfe, *Playing Around*, 36.

8. Zacks, *History Laid Bare*, 300.

INTERLUDE 5

1. lovesherso, http://ourhotwives.org/forum/viewtopic.php?f=8&t=3818
&p=51705&hilit=cervix#p517 (accessed May 11, 2008).

CHAPTER 6

1. D. H. Lawrence, *Lady Chatterley's Lover* (New York: Buccaneer Books, 1983), 17.

2. Lawrence, *Lady Chatterley's Lover*, 41.

3. Lawrence, *Lady Chatterley's Lover*, 42.

4. Lawrence, *Lady Chatterley's Lover*, 51.

5. J. Berens, "The Double Life of Catherine M," *Guardian*, May 19, 2002.

6. P. Popham and E. Murphy, "Tables Turned on the Queen of Promiscuity," *Independent*, August 23, 2008.

7. Isaac Singer, "The House Friend," in *The Death of Methuselah* (New York: Farrar, Strauss and Giroux, 1988), 17.

8. Singer, "The House Friend," 20.

9. Singer, "The House Friend," 24.

10. Polly Vernon, "Love. Sex. Marriage. Affairs," *Observer*, September 7, 2008.

11. Gerald Jacobs, review of *The Act of Love*, by Howard Jacobson, *Telegraph*, September 30, 2008.

12. Doug Sorito, "Penthouse Letters Editor Still Hot for the Job," January 8, 2008, www.thenaughtyamerican.com/index.php/misc/print_version/1221.

13. Kathy Cavanaugh, ed., *Letters to Penthouse XXII: Views from the Top and Bottom* (New York: Time Warner, 2004).

14. mdcucked, http://ourhotwives.org/forum/viewtopic.php?f=5&t=5513&
p=74506&hilit=penthouse+stepfather#p74506 (accessed December 16, 2008).

15. Amber Leigh, *Cuckold* (London: Nexus, 2007), 3.

16. Leigh, *Cuckold*, 107.

17. www.literotica.com/stories/index.php (accessed March 20, 2009).

18. www.ginalanier.com/paranormal relationships (accessed March 20, 2009).

CHAPTER 7

1. Ellis, *Little Essays.*

2. K. Freund, M. Seto, and M. Kuban, "Frotteurism and the Theory of Courtship Disorder," in *Sexual Deviance, Theory, Assessment and Treatment*, ed. D. Richard Laws and William O'Donohue (New York: Guilford Press, 1997), 115.

3. M. Kaplan and R. Krueger, "Psychopathology and Theory," in *Sexual Deviance, Theory, Assessment and Treatment*, ed. D. Richard Laws and William O'Donohue (New York: Guilford Press, 1997), 298

4. Kaplan and Krueger, "Psychopathology," 298.

5. J. Milner and C. Dopke, "Paraphilia Not Otherwise Specified," in *Sexual Deviance, Theory, Assessment and Treatment*, ed. D. Richard Laws and William O'Donohue (New York: Guilford Press, 1997), 416.

6. Milner and Dopke, "Paraphilia," 416.

7. Freund, Seto, and Kuban, "Frotteurism," 115.

8. Milner and Dopke, "Paraphilia," 416.

9. http://www.dshs.state.tx.us/csot/csot_tfacts.shtm (accessed March 20, 2009).

10. Uri Wernik, "The Nature of Explanation in Sexology and the Riddle of Triolism," *Annals of Sex Research* 3, no. 1(1990): 6.

11. Wernik, "Triolism," 8.

12. Wernik, "Triolism," 9.

13. Uri Wernik, personal communication, September 4, 2008.

14. Krafft-Ebing, *Psychopathia Sexualis.*

15. Krafft-Ebing, *Psychopathia Sexualis.*

16. http://www.thestranger.com/seattle/savagelove?oid=115476 (accessed March 20, 2009).

17. http://www.thestranger.com/seattle/savagelove?oid=133984 (accessed March 20, 2009).

18. http://slog.thestranger.com/2007/01/cuckolding_confusion (accessed March 20, 2009).

19. Anonymous, http://ourhotwives.org/forum/ (accessed June 8, 2008).

20. LakeDistrictCouple, http://ourhotwives.org/forum/viewtopic.php?f=6&t=5244&p=79313&hilit=mixed+race+couple#p79313 (accessed January 30, 2009).

21. Ellis, *Little Essays*, 39.

22. Roy Baumeister and Jennifer Butler, "Deviance without Pathology," in *Sexual Deviance, Theory, Assessment and Treatment*, ed. D. Richard Laws and William O'Donohue (New York: Guilford Press, 1997), 231, 236.

23. http://www.hotwivesonline.com (accessed December 10, 2008).

24. http://www.ananova.com/news/story/sm2344515.html (accessed December 10, 2008).

25. http://www.bipolar-lives.com/bipolar-infidelity.html (accessed December 10, 2008).

26. zorro, http://ourhotwives.org/forum/viewtopic.php?f=5&t=5192&p=69959&hilit=authentic#p69959 (accessed November 2, 2008).

27. www.qx.se/english/8655/sweden-to-strike-six-sexual-diagnoses-from-list (accessed March 29, 2009).

28. http://www.ncsfreedom.org/ (accessed March 30, 2009).

CHAPTER 8

1. http://Altlaw.org/v1/cases/532045 (accessed March 20, 2009).

2. http://www.lovemore.com/april/transcript_partner.htm (accessed February 20, 2007).

3. www.courant.com/news/custom/topnews/hcswingerarrests1219.art-dec19.0.6566622.story (accessed February 15, 2009).

4. Dulcie Pearce, "His Kinky Kicks Cost Him Lover," *Sun*, January 17, 2008.

5. www.thelocal.se/14052/20080901 (accessed February 20, 2009).

6. www.msnbc.com/id/24263242/page/2/ (accessed February 20, 2009).

7. R. De Visser, and D. McDonald, "Swing and Roundabouts: Management of Jealousy in Heterosexual Swinging Couples," *British Journal of Social Psychology* 46, no. 2 (2007): 459.

8. Erica Jong, *How to Save Your Own Life* (New York: Holt, Rinehart and Winston, 1977), 47.

9. Ashley Lister, *Swingers* (London: Virgin Books, 2006), 240.

10. Lister, *Swingers*, 242–243.

11. Doc2x, personal communication, September 9, 2008.

INTERLUDE 8

1. Wernik, "Triolism," 12.

CHAPTER 9

1. Klein, *America's War on Sex*, 108.

2. matt2, e-mail to author, September 17, 2008.

3. netflood, http://bb4.redclouds.com//messages/15288957/15288957 .html?1097145655 (accessed January 31, 2008).

4. anonymous, http://bb4.redclouds.com//messages/15288957/15288957 .html?1097145655 (accessed September 16, 2008).

5. Ncal101, e-mail message to the author, September 17, 2008.

6. Husker_hunny, http://bb4.redclouds.com//messages/15288957/ 15288957.html?1097145655 (accessed September 15, 2008).

7. jailmilflover0269, http://bb4.redclouds.com//messages/15288957/ 15288957.html?1097145655 (accessed September 15, 2008).

8. http://sfbay.craigslist.org/cgi-bin/personals.cgi?category=cas (accessed October 13, 2008).

9. www.candymonroe.com (accessed October 25, 2008).

10. www.ultimatecuckold.net (accessed October 15, 2008).

11. www.sagevivant.com/the_cuckold.php (accessed November 15, 2008).

12. http://www.sagevivant.com/quiz.php (accessed October 15, 2008).

13. www.cafepress.com/hotwives (accessed October 15, 2008).

14. www.U|Rockers.com (accessed November 7, 2008).

15. http://www.dogging-info.com (accessed November 7, 2008).

16. Lister, *Swingers*, 53.

17. Lister, *Swingers*, 56.

18. Lister, *Swingers*, 59.

19. Lister, *Swingers*, 63.

20. Lister, *Swingers*, 66.

21. http://groups.yahoo.com/group/naughtykathywillets/ (accessed November 1, 2008).

22. http://www.bigdoggie.net/escorts/by-id/581.html (accessed November 1, 2008).

23. www.turnto23.com/news/9812908/detail .com (accessed March 29, 2009).

24. http://Seattletimes.mwsource.com/html/nationworld/2003250510 _nudephoto08.html (accessed March 29, 2008).

25. http://www.rockymountainnews.com/news/2008/mar/05/cuckold -ex-cop-wife-settle-pueblo-20000/ (accessed March 29, 2008).

26. www.thestranger.com/seattle/savagelove?oid=115476 (accessed March 29, 2008).

27. www.thestranger.com/seattle/savagelove?oid=643679 (accessed March 29, 2008).

INTERLUDE 9

1. Wernik, "Triolism," 12.

CHAPTER 10

1. D. H. Lawrence, *The Rainbow*, http://www.yahooey.comauthors/ lawrence-david-herbert/the-rainbow/chapter-15html.

2. Josephine Lowndes Sevely, *Eve's Secrets, a New Theory of Female Sexuality* (New York: Random House, 1987).

3. www.holisticwisdom.com.

4. Rebecca L. Burch and Gordon G. Gallup Jr., "The Psychobiology of Human Semen," in *Female Infidelity and Paternal Uncertainty*, ed. Platek and Shackelford (New York: Cambridge University Press, 2006), 141–172.

5. phxphun, http://ourhotwives.org/forum/viewtopic.php?f=5&=3284&p =65533&hilit=bareback+gangbang#p65533 (accessed January 22, 2008).

6. Margot, "Cuckold Heaven," in *The Mammoth Book of Women's Erotica*, ed. Sonia Florens (London: Constable & Robinson, 2004), 61–69.

7. Talese, *Thy Neighbor's Wife*, 403.

8. MikeandDeb, http://ourhotwives.org/forum/viewtopic.php?f=6&t =5244&p=79313&hilit=mixed+race+couple#p79313 (accessed November 17, 2008).

9. mdcucked, http://ourhotwives.org/forum/viewtopic.php?f=5&t=4764&p =64737&hilit=cuckolding+taboo#p64737 (accessed January 7, 2008).

10. SoCalCuckold, http://ourhotwives.org/forum/viewtopic.php?f=6&t =5244&p=79339&hilit=cuckolding+taboo#p79339 (accessed January 30, 2009).

11. www.slate.com/id/2154249/ (accessed January 30, 2009).

12. Flaguy, http://bb4.redclouds.com//messages/15288957/15288957 .html?1097145655 (accessed September 14, 2008).

13. docx997x, http://bb4.redclouds.com//messages/15288957/15288957 .html?1097145655 (accessed September 14, 2008).

CHAPTER 11

1. Talese, *Thy Neighbor's Wife*, 599.

2. www.ananova.com/news/story/sm-1697093.html (accessed January 30, 2009).

3. D. Schmitt and D. Buss, "Human Mate Poaching: Tactics and Temptations for Infiltrating Existing Relationships," *Journal of Personality and Social Psychology* 80, no. 6 (2001): 894–917.

4. mdcucked, http://ourhotwives.org/forum/viewtopic.php?f=5&t=5541&p =75103&hilit=love+alpha#p75103 (accessed January 22, 2008).

5. Joann Rodgers, *Sex: A Natural History* (New York: Times Books, 2001), 383.

6. Iris Brent quoted in David Allyn, *Make Love, Not War: The Sexual Revolutions: An Unfettered History* (New York: Routledge, 2001), 225.

7. Fetishfurniturefactory.com (accessed November 1, 2008).

8. Gould, *The Lifestyle*, 208.

9. Gould, *The Lifestyle*, 220–221.

10. Shackelford and Goetz, "Predicting Violence against Women from Men's Mate-retention Behaviors," 65.

SELECTED BIBLIOGRAPHY

Baker, Robin. (1996). *Sperm Wars. Infidelity, Sexual Conflict and Other Bedroom Battles*. New York: Thunder's Mouth Press.

Baumeister, Roy, and Twenge, Jean. (2002). Cultural Suppression of Female Sexuality. *Review of General Psychology* 6, no. 2: 166–203.

Bergner, Daniel. (2009). What Do Women Want? *The New York Times Magazine*, January 22, 2009.

Bergstrand, Curtis, and Williams, Jennifer Blevins. (2000). Today's Alternative Marriage Styles: The Case of Swingers. *Electronic Journal of Human Sexuality* 3 (October): www.ejhs.org/volume3/swing/body.htm.

Black, Wayne. (1967). *A Study of Group Sex in Wife Swapping*. Buffalo, N.Y.: Unique Books.

Blackledge, Catherine. (2004). *The Story of V. A Natural History of Female Sexuality*. New Brunswick, N.J.: Rutgers University Press.

Brasch, R. (1995). *How Did Sex Begin? The Sense and Nonsense of Sexual Customs and Traditions*. Sydney, Australia: HarperCollins Publishers.

Buss, David. (1994). *The Evolution of Desire. Strategies of Human Mating*. New York: Basic Books.

Carneiro, Robert. "Kuikuru." Available online at: www.everyculture.com/South-America/Kuikuru.html.

Cavanaugh, Kathy. (2004). *Letters to Penthouse XXII: Views From Top and Bottom*. New York: Time Warner.

Duckworth, J., and Levitt, E. (1985). Personality Analysis of a Swingers' Club. *Lifestyles* 8, no. 1(fall): 35–45.

Easton, D., and Liszt, C. (1997). *The Ethical Slut: Guide to Infinite Sexual Possibilities*. San Francisco: Greenery Press.

Falk, Candace. (1990). *Love, Anarchy, and Emma Goldman*. New Brunswick, N.J.: Rutgers University Press. Available online at www.questia.com.

Fisher, Helen (1992). *Anatomy of Love. The Natural History of Monogamy, Adultery, and Divorce*. New York: W. W. Norton.

——. (2004). *Why We Love. The Nature and Chemistry of Romantic Love*. New York: Henry Holt.

Florens, Sonia. (2004). *The Mammoth Book of Women's Erotic Fantasies*. London: Constable & Robinson.

Fonseca, Claudia. (2001). "Philanderers, Cuckold, and Wily Women, A Reexamination of Gender Relations in a Brazilian Working-class Neighborhood." *Men and Masculinities* 3, no. 3: 261–277.

Gould, Terry. (2000). *The Lifestyle, A Look at the Erotic Rites of Swingers*. Buffalo, N.Y.: Firefly.

Groneman, Carol. (2000). *Nymphomania, A History*. New York: W. W. Norton.

Heinlein, Robert A. (1961). *Stranger in a Strange Land*. New York: Putnam.

Herek, G. (2004). "Beyond 'Homophobia': Thinking about Sexual Prejudice and Stigma in the Twenty-first Century." *Sexuality Research and Social Policy Journal of NSRC* 1, no. 2: 6–24.

——. (2000). "The Psychology of Sexual Prejudice." *Current Directions in Psychological Science* 9: 19–22.

Heyn, Dalma. (1992). *The Erotic Silence of the American Wife*. New York: Turtle Bay.

Jacobson, Howard. (2009). *Act of Love*. New York: Simon and Schuster.

Janus, S., and Janus, C. (1993). *The Janus Report on Sexual Behavior*. New York: Wiley.

Jenks, Richard. (1998). "Swinging: A Review of the Literature." *Archives of Sexual Behavior* 27, no. 5: 507–521.

Jones, James H. (1997). *Alfred C. Kinsey, A Public/Private Life*. New York: W. W. Norton.

Kessler, R., et al. (2005). "Prevalence and Treatment of Mental Disorders, 1990 to 2003." *New England Journal of Medicine* 352, no. 24: 2515–2523.

Kinsey, Alfred, Pomeroy, Wardell, and Martin, Clyde. (1953). *Sexual Behavior of the Human Male*. Philadelphia: W. B. Saunders.

Kinsey, Alfred, Pomeroy, Wardell, Martin, Clyde, and Gebhardt, Paul, et al. (1953). *Sexual Behavior of the Human Female*. Philadelphia: W. B. Saunders.

Klein, Marty. (2008). *America's War on Sex, The Attack on Law, Lust, and Liberty*. Westport, Conn.: Praeger.

Kraft-Ebing, Richard von. *Psychopathia Sexualis With Especial Reference to the Antipathic Sexual Instinct A Medico-Forensic Study*. Available online at: www.archive.org/details/psychopathiasexu00krafuoft.

LaSala, M. C. (2004). "Extradyadic Sex and Gay Male Couples: Comparing Monogamous and Nonmonogamous Relationships." *Families in Society: The Journal of Contemporary Social Services* 85, no. 3: 405–412.

Laumann, E., Gagnon, J., Michael, R., and Michaels, S. (1994). *The Social Organization of Sexuality: Sexual Practices in the United States*. Chicago: University of Chicago Press.

Laws, D. Richard, and O'Donohue, William. (1997). *Sexual Deviance, Theory, Assessment and Treatment*. New York: Guilford Press.

Leigh, Amber. (2007). *Cuckold*. London: Nexus.

Lister, Ashley. (2006). *Swingers. True Confessions from Today's Swinging Scene*. London: Virgin Books.

Lowndes Sevely, Josephine. (1987). *Eve's Secrets, A New Theory of Female Sexuality*. New York: Random House.

Masters, William H., Johnson, Virginia E., and Kolodny, Robert C. (1994). *Heterosexuality*. New York: HarperCollins.

———. (1988). *Masters and Johnson on Sex and Human Loving*. Boston: Little, Brown.

McCullough, Derek, and Hall, David S. (2003). "Polyamory—What It Is and What It Isn't." *Electronic Journal of Human Sexuality* 6 (February) at: www.ejhs.org/volume6/polyamory.htm.

McLean, Kirsten. (2004). "Negotiating (Non)Monogamy: Bisexuality and Intimate Relationships." *Journal of Bisexuality* 4, no. 1: 55–82.

Muller-Lyer, F. (1930). *Evolution of Modern Marriage, A Sociology of Sexual Relations*. Translated by Isabella C. Wigglesworth. New York: Alfred A. Knopf.

Nichols, M., and Shernoff, M. (2007). "Therapy with Sexual Minorities, Queering Practice," in *Principles and Practice of Sex Therapy*. 4th ed. Edited by Sandra Leiblum. New York: Guilford Press.

Pallotta-Chiarolli, M., and Lubowitz, S. (2003). "'Outside belonging': Multi-sexual Relationships as Border Existence." *Journal of Bisexuality* 3, no. 1: 53–85.

Partridge, Burgo. (2005). *A History of Orgies*. 1958. Reprint, London: Sevenoaks.

Pearce, Dulcie. (2008). "His Kinky Kicks Cost Him Lover." The *Sun*, at: www.thesun.co.uk/sol/homepage/woman/real_life/article695973.ece.

Platek, Steven, and Shackelford, Todd. (2006). *Female Infidelity and Paternal Uncertainty, Evolutionary Perspectives on Male Anti-Cuckoldry Tactics*. New York: Cambridge University Press.

Prioleau, Elizabeth. (2004). *Seductress: Women who Ravished the World and Their Lost Art of Love*. New York: Penguin.

Quaife, G. R. (1979). *Wanton Wenches and Wayward Wives: Peasants and Illicit Sex in Early Seventeenth Century England*. New Brunswick, N.J.: Rutgers University Press.

Roach, Mary. (2008). *Bonk. The Curious Coupling of Science and Sex*. New York: W. W. Norton.

Rodgers, Joann. (2001). *Sex, A Natural History*. New York: Times Books.

Rubin, R. (2001). "Alternative Lifestyles Revisited, or Whatever Happened to Swingers, Group Marriages, and Communes?" *Journal of Family Issues* 22, no. 6: 711–726.

Rust, P. C. (1996). "Monogamy and Polyamory: Relationship Issues for Bisexuals." In *Bisexuality: The Psychology and Politics of an Invisible Minority*. Edited by B. Firestein. Thousand Oaks, Calif.: Sage Publications.

Shand-Tucci, Douglas. (1997). *The Art of Scandal, The Life and Times of Isabella Stewart-Gardner*. New York: HarperCollins.

Sheff, E. (2005). "Polyamorous Women, Sexual Subjectivity and Power." *Journal of Contemporary Ethnography* 34, no. 3: 251–283.

Shernoff, M. (2000). "Case Studies: Monogamy and Gay Men." *Family Therapy Networker* (March/April) at: www.findarticles.com.

Singer, Isaac. (1988). *The Death of Methuselah and Other Stories*. New York: Farrar, Strauss, and Giroux.

Talese, Gay. (1980). *Thy Neighbor's Wife*. New York: Dell.

Vernon, Polly. (2008). "Love. Sex. Marriage. Affairs." *The Observer*, at: www.guardian.co.uk/lifeandstyle/2008/sep/07/relationships.women.

Vivant, Sage. (2007). *Your Erotic Personality: Identifying and Understanding Your Sexual Self*. New York: Penguin.

Wallace, Hugh. (1997). *Another Way: Beyond Sexual Monogamy*, at: www.sexcellence.info.

Wallace, Irving. (1971). *The Nympho and Other Maniacs*. New York: Simon and Schuster.

Walston, Jasmine. (2001). Polyamory: An Exploratory Study of Responsible Multi-Partnering. Unpublished research study conducted at Indiana University Southeast, under the advisement of Richard Jenks, PhD, Professor of Sociology. Obtained from the author. Available in the Kinsey Institute Library, Polyamory Collection.

Weber, S. (2002). "Survey Results: Who are We and Other Interesting Impressions." *Loving More* 30 (summer).

Weiner-Davis, Michele. (2008). *The Sex-Starved Wife: What to Do When He's Lost Desire*. New York: Simon and Schuster.

Weitzman, Geri. (1999). What Psychology Professionals Should Know About Polyamory: The Lifestyles and Mental Health Concerns of Polyamorous Individuals. Based on a paper presented at the 8th Annual Diversity Conference, March 12, 1999, Albany, N.Y., at: www.polyamory.org/~joe/polypaper.htm.

Wernik, Uri. (1990). "The Nature of Explanation in Sexology and the Riddle of Triolism." *Annals of Sex Research* 3, no. 1: 5–20.

Wolf, Naomi. (1997). *Promiscuities*. New York: Random House.

Wolfe, Leanna. (2003). Jealousy and Transformation in Polyamorous Relationships. Dissertation at: drleannaWolfe.com/Dissertation.pdf.

Wolfe, Linda. (1975). *Playing Around: Women and Extramarital Sex*. New York: William Morrow.

Yalom, Marilyn. (2001). *A History of the Wife*. New York: HarperCollins.

Zacks, Richard. (1994). *History Laid Bare: Love, Sex, and Perversity from the Ancient Romans to Warren G. Harding*. New York: HarperCollins.

INDEX